We Had a Life:
My Years at Kalaupapa

By Cathrine Puahala

Edited By Charles Langlas

Pili Productions
Hilo, Hawai'i 2016

Frontispiece

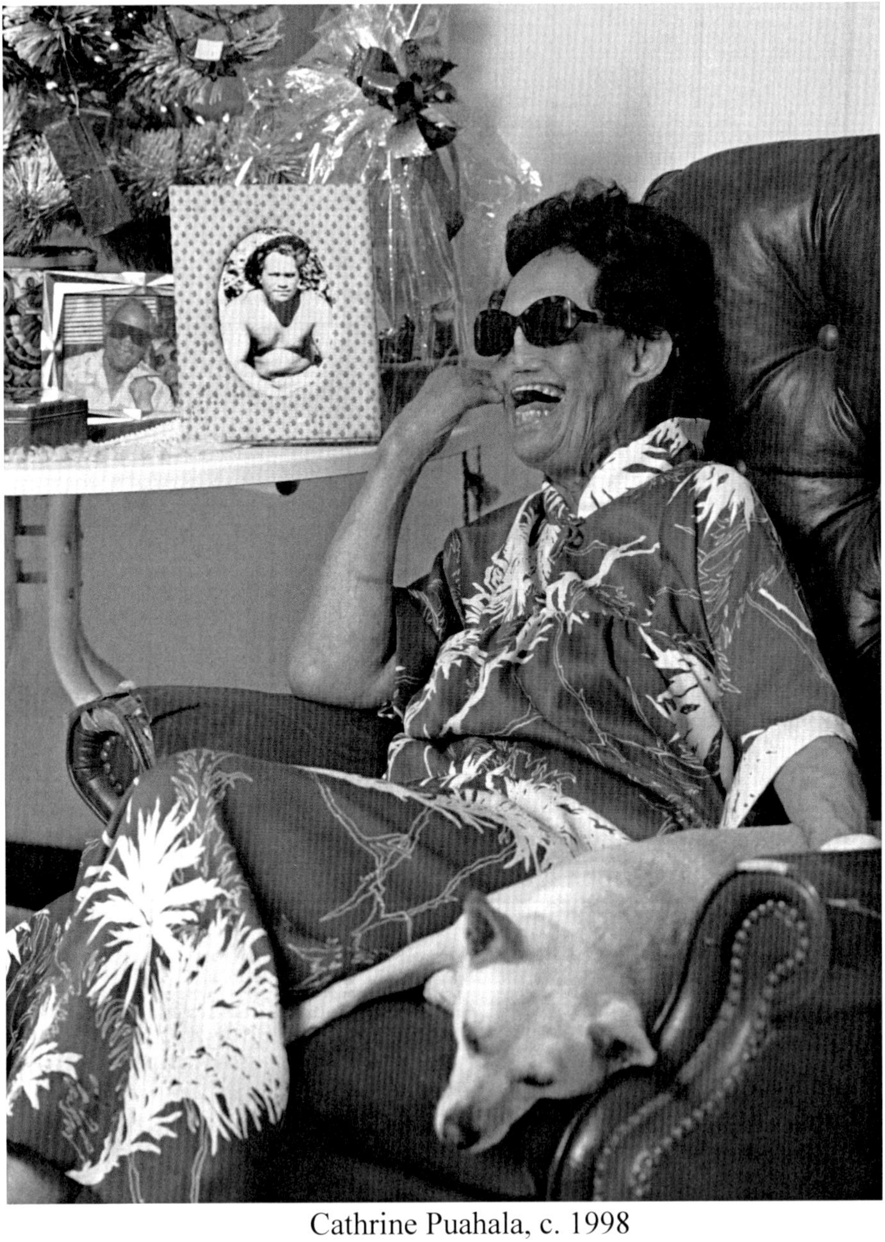

Cathrine Puahala, c. 1998
(photo by Shuzo Uemoto)

Preface

I came to Kalaupapa in 2001 as a cultural anthropologist, hired by the National Park Service, along with my colleagues Ka'ohulani McGuire and Sonia Juvik, to study the Kalaupapa community, which lies on an isolated peninsula below the towering cliffs of the north shore of Moloka'i, Hawai'i. Specifically we were to study the relationships between the Hansen's Disease patients at Kalaupapa and the "kokuas," the State Department of Health workers who provide support services to the patients and workers of the Kalaupapa National Historical Park who maintain the park. (In accordance with state policy and patient preference, we use the term Hansen's disease, rather than the older term leprosy, which has pejorative connotations.)

In the process of interviewing the patients, we quickly became enamored of one colorful woman, Cathrine Puahala, a fascinating raconteur, who tells her story in this book. When we met Cathrine, she was living alone with her dog Sunday, since her husband had died four years earlier. She was determined to stay in her own house even though she had a number of disabilities common among the older Hansen's disease patients at Kalaupapa who did not receive the antibiotic sulphone drugs in time to prevent the ravages of the disease. She was almost completely blind, had limited use of her hands because her fingers had atrophied, and had lost sensation in her hands as well. Still, she valued and insisted on her independence.

But Cathrine did not let her physical disabilities stand in her way. She kept up with current news of the nation and the world by watching the televised news on CNN. In spite of spending most of her days at home, she always seemed to know everything that was going on at Kalaupapa. Once the policy of segregating the patients was ended in 1969, she traveled a good deal. Beginning in 1997, she got involved with IDEA, the International Organization for Integration, Dignity and

Economic Advancement, an organization formed to work for the human rights and welfare of Hansen's disease patients. She made four trips overseas on behalf of IDEA—to Spain, China, New York, and Japan. She also traveled to Belgium with several other patients for the premier of the movie "Molokai: The Story of Father Damien," which had been filmed at Kalaupapa. While we knew her, she flew to Honolulu periodically and went to shops and restaurants. She loved to shop for clothes and accessories at the second-hand store next to Hale Mohalu[1]. Once or twice a year she went to Las Vegas for a few days to gamble and to take in the shows. In 2006, she decided to start spending her nights at the Kalaupapa Care Home, but she still went home to her own house every morning and spent the day there.

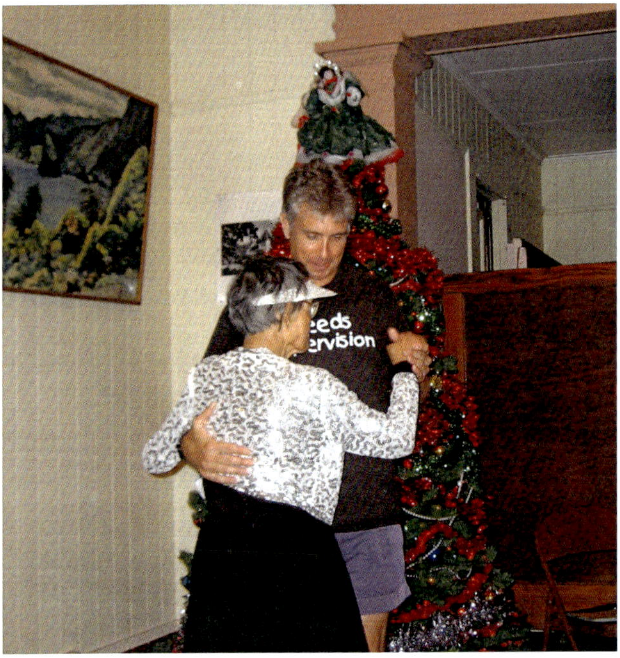

Cathrine, dancing with Eric at New Year's Eve party, 2006. (photo by C. Langlas)

[1] Hale Mohalu is a facility for Hansen's disease Patients in Honolulu, established in 1949 when the Kalihi Hospital facility in Honolulu was closed (see p. 96). In recent years, the patients who live at Kalaupapa have stayed there when they need medical treatment unavailable at Kalaupapa.

Cathrine loved parties and when she went partying, she wanted to drink. She also loved to dress up. Despite her limited vision, she kept a stylish wardrobe and carefully chose her clothes and accessories. She loved color and glitter. Her trademark was to wear a visor both daytime and evening. When she wore a slinky silver and black gown for New Years Eve, she had a visor with rhinestones to wear with it. Her artistic flair also showed in the crafts she undertook.

For many years when she could still use her hands, she sewed clothes, strung seed leis, made flower leis for May Day celebrations and constructed decorative Christmas trees. When she could no longer do those things herself, she directed her housekeeper in making competition entries for her.

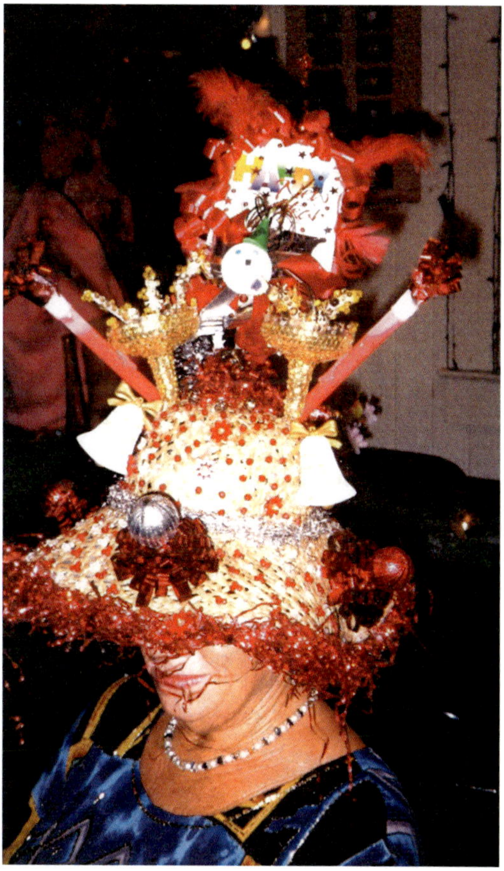

Nurse Julie Sigler in electrified hat made for New Year‘s Eve hat contest, 2006. (photo by Ka‘ohulani McGuire)

In her last years of life, Cathrine decided that there wasn't enough happening in Kalaupapa. In 2006, she sponsored a hat contest for the New Year's Eve party. People came with fabulously crafted hats. The contest was won by a woman in a hat with light bulbs that lit up.

Cathrine also loved food. She had been a good cook of local food, but after she became blind she had to stop cooking. Since she had lost sensation in her hands, she could neither feel nor see if her hands were getting seriously burned. So she relied on others to cook for her, me included, and she made sure that the food was cooked right—her way. She would say, "Going add shoyu, yeah? Two table-spoon," or "Be sure fry the fish crisp." Once she requested that we make her palusami, a Samoan dish made of lūʻau (taro) leaves, coconut milk and corned beef. She loved my daughter's éclairs that I brought when I visited, saying "Tell your daughter the éclair was eaten with care."

I have left Cathrine's story as she told it, mostly in Hawaiian Creole English, locally referred to as "Pidgin," because I want for you to "hear" her masterful voice, in all its color and richness, rather than change it into Standard English prose, and because it is the preferred mode of story-telling among local folks. Like many local English speakers, Cathrine code-switches sometimes from Pidgin to Standard English grammatical construction. For example, she says "we'd grown up together," instead of using the Pidgin construction, "we wen grow up together." Likewise, she switches back and forth between the Standard English "kind" and the Pidgin version "kine."

For additional background on Kalaupapa to help in understanding Cathrine's story, see the appendix, which describes the changes to Kalaupapa Settlement over time and describes Kalaupapa Peninsula as a place during the time that Cathrine was alive.

Themes

A number of themes stand out in Cathrine's story that need contextualization. Two of them appear in the prologue, including the title theme, "we had a life." Cathrine speaks often of how the life the patients lived at Kalaupapa from the 1940s to the 1960s was good, of how they lived just like people elsewhere. The historical context of this theme is that the sulphone drugs came in the 1940s. Prior to that people often died young and perhaps life was not so good for patients at Kalaupapa. But the years when Cathrine grew up and married at Kalaupapa were good ones for her and the other patients. More recently, life at Kalaupapa has become less good, because the group of patients has gotten too small to support the social life of the community.

Another theme of the prologue is that Hansen's disease is not contagious. Cathrine says this a couple of times in the material that has been put together for this book. I have often heard her and other patients say it in conversation. It reflects both what doctors have told them and their own observation of people exposed to Hansen's disease over a long time. Some who are exposed to the disease develop symptoms and others never do, because it depends on their immune system. At the same time, Cathrine says that the disease came to her and her siblings from her father's cousin. It is easy to oversimplify what is a complex phenomenon. It remains the case that Hansen's disease is contagious: *Mycobaterium leprae*, which causes the symptoms of Hansen's disease, can pass from those who have it in its most active form (lepromatous) to others. Those who are exposed to the bacterium may or may not develop Hansen's disease symptoms, depending on their immune system. Some of those who are exposed to the bacterium will be immune, some will develop a less serious form of Hansen's disease (tuberculoid), and others a more serious form (lepromatous). If the bacteria are not suppressed by drugs, individuals with the lepromatous form develop much more severe symptoms and are much more likely to infect others than are those with the tuberculoid form.

Another matter that needs contextualization is Cathrine's talk about drinking. For many years, most of the patients at Kalaupapa were heavy drinkers. It is not difficult to see why. In the days before the sulphone drugs came, drink was a refuge for many from the desperate knowledge of their early death. Partying and drinking became a way of life at Kalaupapa and it continued as a main form of recreation after the coming of the sulphone drugs. As Cathrine says, she joined in that partying so that her husband wouldn't be going out without her. By the time we got to Kalaupapa in 2001, there was much less drinking. Most of the patients had health problems and had given up regular drinking for that reason. Cathrine, too, drank mainly on special occasions.

Charles Langlas, editor

Prologue

We are the same like outside people. You know? We no different, only that our features look different. I hope people will read the story and think of what really happened, how we lived, what kind shenanigans went on. Because it's natural. Look at Peyton Place. We lived just like other people outside. Only that we are so well protected by the state.

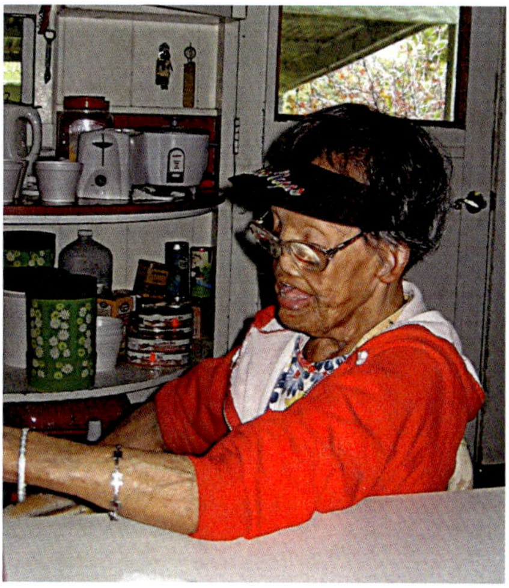

Cathrine, 2008.
(photo by C. Langlas)

People on the outside only knows of our life here is handed out to us on a silver platter, you know? They don't think we have a life here, but we do. We live just as good as they are, you know. Life is good here. I don't wanta live anyplace else in this world but Kalaupapa. It's my home. I would like to live here and die here. And be buried here.

When we first came to Kalaupapa, all you saw was flowers growing along side of the road and the trees just full with blossoms. Lots of plants, iron wood trees, and night blooming cereus--they were all on the stonewall blooming beautiful. They had a lot of nice purple bougainvillea. It went up alongside of the road. It went all the way up and when it was in bloom, it was so pretty, so beautiful. And up at Staff Row, you see the trees all lined up, the yellow shower, the pink shower—all in May. The month of May, it's just full with flowers. Covered, the whole tree. And there's a lot of bees. When we pass by, we can hear the bees (bzzz), and we use to love watch them because they go in every flower and jumping to the next. When we came and we just walking up the road, all you smell is plumerias, the fragrance of flowers.

We are so lucky to have the mountains and the ocean, there's two. This place was made perfect for us. I don't think we would have been happier in any other place. I think God made it so that we had everything. We have the beautiful mountains. And then when you tired look at the mountain, look at the ocean. And you go Kalawao, Kalawao is a beautiful spot. You know when you stay at the Old Baldwin Home and you look out to the two islands? It is just perfect. I don't think there's any other place as beautiful as Kalawao.

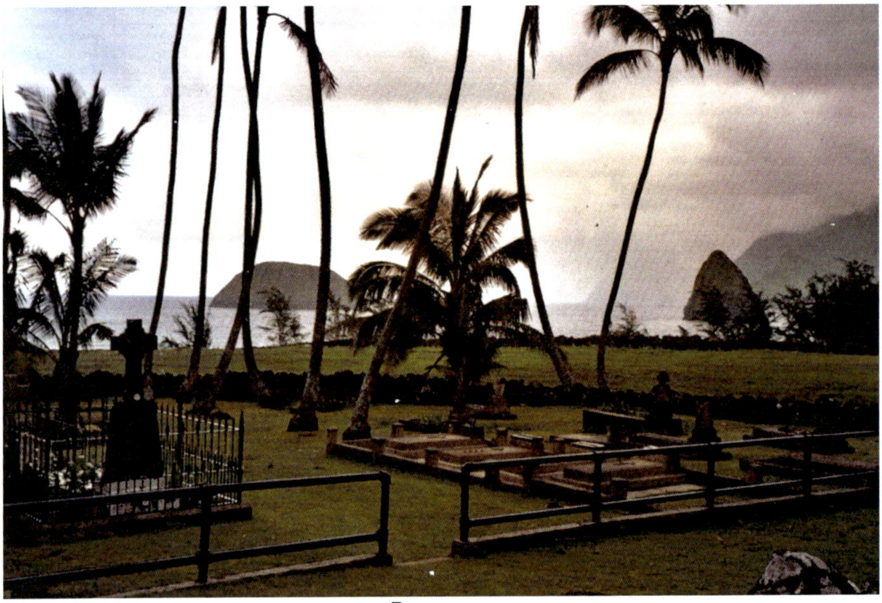

Mōkapu and ʻŌkala Islands from Kalawao.
(photo by C. Langlas)

So this is my home. And I hope they will never tell us to leave. That will kill a lot of us. But now we don't know what's in store for us. Because we're only down to 42, I think [as of 2002]. We don't know what they're gonna do now. Sometime there's talk about handing us over to the people at Pearl City. All I know is the National Park was willing to let us stay here. A lot of us say, if they let us stay here, if we gotta pay our own electricity, water, or carpentry work, plumber job, maybe we gotta pay that out of our own pockets, you know? So we don't know what's going to happen in the years ahead.

There're some people still afraid [of us]. But at least they're more friendly to us [now]. We can see the change. Used to be, when we used to walk, the people would go far away from us, like we scare them because of the disease. And the doctors are to be blamed for that. They got the people scared out at Kalihi Hospital. Yeah. They got our family scared. See there was a fence it was a barrier that you cannot go over, they cannot come in. That was for, like off-limits. And then when they saw the family embracing over this one fence, they build another fence, to separate us farther away. We couldn't stretch over because they made it far enough where you cannot embrace anymore. They were the ones that frighten our family, those in authority. And only to find out now that this sick is not contagious; it's an individual species. We come from the same mother and father, my sister and I. She didn't get it. They say your sister was very strong. It went for her, only it cannot. She was able to fight it. I had three sisters outside--same father, same mother—and they didn't get it. But we were—our immune system had broken down, unable to fight, so we were the unlucky ones. We got the sick.

Chapter 1. Getting the Disease (1927 to 1941)

I was born 1927. When my mother died, I think I was about four almost five. And I think I had the disease already. I had the disease when I was three I think. My hands was swollen. I grew up in Pauoa Valley and I went to Pauoa School. But when I go school, the teacher asked me, "How come your hands like that?" I say I drink plenty milk. But they never know I had the sick.

My father was Solomon Kuahine. The disease is on my father's side. Because my cousin's mother—that's my father's first cousin—that's where the disease start. Only me and my sister Eunice got the disease, with my brothers Samson, Ah Wah, and my youngest brother Chuck. My sister Agnes, she never had the disease. But she got other kind sick—asthma, heart, after my mother. My mother left us all with some kind of problem. She's a sickly person. I think my father and her shouldn't have married. The immune system was no good. I think my father should have married one Portagee or something else. The immune system would be different, not all on the Hawaiian. It'd be stronger. But who knows.

Who I remember at home was just my sister Agnes, my sister Eunice I think, and then me, then Ku'ulei, and then Chuckie. My two older brothers went in Kalihi Hospital almost about the same time. But I was younger then, I didn't realize, I didn't get to look at them like they were my brothers. I used to go down to visit my two brothers and my sister. And my brother Samson, he had the raspy voice and I cannot understand. They talk like "hah-hah-hah [hoarsely]," you know, like that, uh? Because he had a tube in his throat to help him breathe. I used to ask my father, "How come my brother talk like that?" But you see Hawaiian people, they never give you an explanation. I ask, "Papa, how come brother talk like that?" And he just shut me up. "Be quiet." He don't want me asking questions.

That's why we don't grow up to know a lotta things. Your father and mother don't tell you. They think you don't need to know. Yeah? That's how. That's the only time I asked for my brother.

And then when we went back again, they were gone. I think that's the last time we was supposed to see them. The two of them came out to Kalaupapa together, the two brothers. My sister stayed back at Kalihi. Then my sister Eunice went. But I tell you, if the medicine was there that day, I think all of us live. But there was no medicine. It was not the right time. They come the wrong time. They are sacrifice for us.

So I went in to see the doctor. We all went, the whole family. When we get family in here, they used to corral the whole family. Not the outside cousin, the immediate family only—mother, father, sister, brother. They corral all us and we are made to go examine. And they examine all the kids first. That's how they saw a white spot on my backside. So the doctors always feel that there's something there. So they get the razor blade, and they squeeze the tissue so you won't feel it, and they sort of scrape some tissue up, some blood, you know. Then they put it on the glass and under the microscope. That's how they saw the bug. They told my father that I had to go in Kalihi, that I had the germ. People are more afraid of this germ, because they say it's contagious. You saw that boy that was down here? He's married to a patient, and yet, he never got the disease. It is not contagious. The doctor said that for us be more careful, you know? But it was not right for us to be thought of as contagious.

I had a feeling I had something, but they don't tell me outright. So much secret! I used to wonder why my father separate me from my brother and sister. They were younger than me. Always he drop me off in the country—Kaneohe, Ka'alaea, my father's mother and father. Those days we call them tutu lady and tutu man. My father took me down there quite often. I preferred it down there anyway. I can go swimming, I can go crabbing. 1935 was the best year I stayed down there. Cause you put the crab net down, and the water is waist high.

You could see the crab crawling in to the bait. Yeah. You cannot see that today. And then my grandmother making charcoal for the iron. Once a week they iron, yeah? So my grandmother makin all the charcoal. And she tell me for throw the net in the water. So I let the net go down, and I watch, and I can see. Crabs were big before. Now they like that [small]. No more the kind officer to check on people, to stop fishing, or catching the young one. No more that kind now. So I catch 'em, then I say, "Tutu, get five." "Oh, nough, nough. Pull 'em up." My grandmother throw 'em in the hot coal. Ohhhh, I really scared because they alive, you know. But because she gonna eat it, it's okay. But not to torture them. So that's all we eat. That's enough lunch.

My father always separated us. And later on I found out why, because they think I had the disease. My fingers were all straight, but all swollen. He probably knew that I had the disease, because I had two brothers and a sister in here already. I'd be the fourth one. He was almost like hiding me from that guy, Kikila. That's his last name. He was a bounty hunter like. He work for the Board the Health. I don't think there is a name Kikila in the telephone book. I think that whole family was wiped out. A lotta Hawaiians cursed that name. So that's the one always been looking for people for bring inside here. And he left a line of broken hearts. You know, family crying, children crying. He pure Hawaiian. But the money was good. Ten dollars a head. So I guess that's how.

I was at Pauoa School. I went to school six years old, I went kindergarten. And then six, seven, eight, I went second grade. Then I skip, they put me in third grade. Just like, the lesson was kinda easy so I just went one grade higher. I think I would have been a smart girl. I was one that caught on fast. And I was in the 3rd grade, I was eight I think, my hands was swollen already. But the children never thought about anything with me. It's the grownups that start whispering, yeah? They look at me and they whisper. Then, just before school was out, my father had a letter not to bring me back school again, to go see the Board of Health after.

They took me outta school. I didn't know why. But they said going be vacation time, so you don't have to come back. So that's what I thought, vacation. And then my father told me I don't have to go back school. And I just hung around home, nothing to do. So I took this long walks to town. I did all kind—go up the ice house, watch 'em how they cut the ice. They did all the shavings. You go there, eat the shaving, just like shave ice. But, you know, get the oil taste. Yeah.

My young life was real lonesome. I don't know why I was chosen to be like that, alone at a very young age, but I was always by myself. When my mother died I had nobody. My sister Agnes went to school, my father went to work, my brother Chuckie and sister Kuʻulei was at the neighbor's house. And I think my father wanted to keep them away from me. I was home alone, so I was free to do and go where I wanted. As if nobody cared, you know? So I learned how to walk down the road. And I do this all the time and I come back, so I know the road how to come home. And each time I go a little bit farther away, until I got to see Princess Theater and Fort Street. From Pauoa I walked downtown Honolulu. And I go in the Kress store and look at all the nice things. No more money, you know. I just look all around, pick up the things, put 'em back. Then I walk out, because I know already I not supposed to take anything, that policeman was goin' catch me. I smell all the food, but no money, so I walk home. And was no problem at all. I had fun! And I got home, and just in back of that my father came home. I run and say, "Hello Papa." He say, "Hello." I go by him and then I watch what he doing, fixing this, fixing that. And then I took another road, I went to Queen's Hospital on Punchbowl Road. I learn how to go that way. That's how I know Honolulu. Till today I know where to go. And I know all the rivers when they come down. I picture them in my mind, where it's going to. And it goes out to River Street, and it goes out to Alawai Canal, all the different area. I study all that when I was a little girl. I was really akamai [smart] for one small kid. I don't tell my father where I went. He's going tell me not to, baimby get lost. Cannot get lost. Once you know the street, you know the rest.

But they fed me the idea that I was goin back to school, cause he took me shopping. He bought about four dresses, and two slips, shoes, and a sweater. So I think, oh, I going back school. But no, he was getting me ready for Kalihi Hospital. Aunty Kapeka, she even took me to Kawaiha'o Church when I was eight years old. She make me sit by the altar for ask God for spare me, cause she knew I would be going to Kalihi Hospital. So she took me to the altar and made me sleep all night over there. She wen stay there with me. And had the other families too, they all slept there. And she prayed all kine. I think so, other families used to do that. 'As[2] the last hope, yeah? And they pray for me all night. We stayed until 5:00 in the morning. She never get answer. She left Kawaiaha'o; she joined the Kaumakapili Church. She was angry.

Then Papa put all these things in a small little basket suitcase. And I was wondering what's going on. I say, "Papa, I going school, yeah?" "No, no, no. You not going to school." Well, then one day he took me on this ride. I was wondering why he was so nice that day. He took me to E.K. Fernandes show. He never take my brother and my sister, only me. Jus like the "Last Hurrah" or something. I going to go all this places, cause I not gonna do it again.

And then one day he helped me get a bath, change clothes, and then he took me to the car. Inside is the little bag. I look at him and say, "Where we going, Papa?" He don't say nothing. Back up the car, going all the way. And I remember the places that we was passing, that was my auntie's house at Dillingham Boulevard. I say, "Oh, this Auntie's house." He say, "Yeah." We passed that, and then we pass Oahu Prison, going down that long drive. And I said, "Oh, this is where Brother is." My brother Ah Wah and Samson was in there. They were patients, but they were gone already, they went to Kalaupapa. He don't say nothing. He park the car by the nurses' quarters. Then he

---

[2] 'As: this is the pidgin version of "that's."

reach for me, my hand. I grab his arm. He helped me down from the car. I walk inside with him. I look at him and I look at my suitcase. I was getting scared already. I start crying. And we reached the door, there's a pear tree [avocado], that's where everybody separate, by the statue. If the statue could talk, it would tell us all the crys that he heard—from children, from mothers gave birth that have to be separated, from men. Even men cry. It was a sad place. Then I saw the nurse coming. Oh, I start screaming already. "Papa, we go Papa, we go." He say, "No, you stay here." Soon as she grabbed my hand, I screamed. I grab my father's leg, I hang on. He took off my hand, he say, "You go with the nurse." I hold on, hold on. He try to take my fingers off, yeah? And the nurse tell me, "Cmon, let's go inside." I say, "No, no." And then my father took my hand loose. He look at me, he say, "You go inside with the nurse." I just scream my head off. And while he was going out, he had his head down. I yell for him. "Papa." He never turn around and look at me. I know my father was crying. It hurts seeing one of your child get taken away. He never turned around. And he went in the car, he left. The nurse told me, "Cmon, let's go."

And then I smell the hospital. You can tell hospital, they have a certain smell, you know. Oh, I didn't wanta go in there. But I went in. They make me take a bath and change into the pajamas. Oh, I cried in the hospital. And I went into my bed. I didn't wanta eat. I was broken-hearted. And different patients came to my room, tried to talk to me. Say, "Don't worry. You'll get well and go home." And the doctor told me when he came, he said, "You'll be here six months, you can go home." That wasn't true. I'm here sixty years in this kind place. And now this is my home. I don't wanta go home; I wanta stay here. I been separated too long. My family is just like strangers. They want to see me, but it's not the same when I go home. It's not the same.

I feel like being taken to Kalihi really broke up a lotta things that I could have been, I could have done. That was taken away from me. Cause after I was about seven, my father took me to the country to live with grandmother. I always stayed there, you know, so my grandmother was teachin me Hawaiian. I would have been good at it because that's all she spoke. And I would have learned. Children learn faster. And what I feel was taken away from me—my life, I could speak Hawaiian. I lost that. I never speak Hawaiian ever again. Too old.

Kalihi Hospital, at first like a dull place. It was not exciting. If not for the children I don't know what would happen. The children was there, we always went out to the swing to play. The boys live in the front building, the girls live in the back building. And we all play together. And that kinda took our mind off our family, you know. That's why when my father took me in, they told my father not to come back for a whole month. Because they wanted us to get used to. If you see them once, start crying. So my father stayed away for the whole month. And by the time he came back to see me, I was so busy playing with the kids that I didn't miss him anymore. So when they said, "Cathrine, you have visitor at the line," I say, "Ohhhh." You know, I was playin hide and seek, and you know kids. So I walk up there, I said, "Hello Papa." Not like I was the first time [when he left me there]. And he said, "How are you?" You know, we talk like that. And there was only one fence separating us. And then because some people they hug the family, they made two fence to keep us apart. And we couldn't hug anymore, we just could touch the hand. Not supposed to, we sneak. Because somebody's always watching us. They see us hugging, they would come on the loudspeaker, and then, "Do not touch." They make us feel so bad, you know.

We were children then, yeah? We got up early in the morning. 4:00. And the boys and the girls all stuck together. We just like brothers and sisters. Because Sarah[3] took care of us, girls and boys both, for only $5 a month. We get together, say where we going this morning. We're gonna go over the fence, and we're goin up the road,

---

[3] Sarah Meier was a young woman patient at Kalihi who was given the job of caring for a group of young boys and girls there.

and we like pick flowers. You know, so the boys pick flowers for their room. All comin with flowers in our hands. And then we go home to the room, put flowers in the vase, and then we just sing. After that we get together and we go down, there's a hau tree that just hung over like. And we all sat on the tree. We were innocent children. You know, just like we were family together, the boys and the girls. And we talk story, all kindsa story.

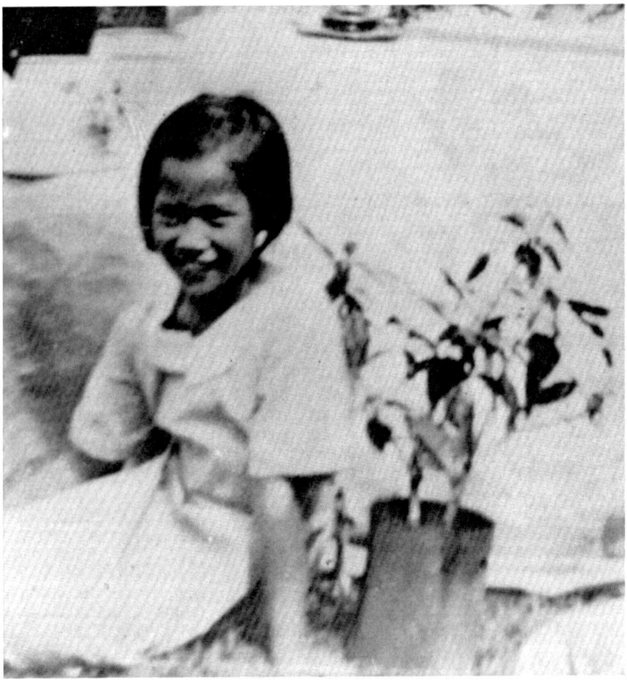

Cathrine at Kalihi Hospital, c. 1938. (photographer unknown)

They used to have movie chapters [serials]. Flash Gordon. Every Monday and Friday we had the chapters. And we won't miss that, because get Flash Gordon inside. He was [played by] Buster Crabbe, and he was young. He could have been 19, 20 years old. He was very good. And then all us young kids went imitate what we see in the movie. So we get together in the evening after supper. We were sitting on the grass—there must have been twenty of us—and we said, "What you going do tonight?" They said, "Let's play Flash Gordon." Then they said, "I be Dr. Zhakov, I be Princess Margie, I be Ming," you know. They always want to act the part. Then we said, "I'll be the stone man." And we make all the sounds that we hear on the screen. Stand against the wall, and get somebody bust up, we come outta the wall, makin the sounds and grab 'em. And you know, we had so much fun doing that. Then they said, "What we gonna do tomorrow?" And they say, "Let's do John Hall and that story down Pagopago side." It's a South Pacific. We dance the hula. We make hula skirt with the coconut fronds. We just sew 'em roughly, you know. Down around our waist. And we put flower in our hair. And we dare who going be John Hall, who going be the main girl. We just do things ourself. We keep ourself busy.

School started in the morning, 8:00, with the raising of the flag. Pledge allegiance and then school start. And then about 10:00, we go in the back room and the teacher play piano. He get right hand lōlō [paralyzed], this one. I think he had the sick before. And he used to sound good. He only play one hand, bass and soprano. And then I listen up. And then we go in the class again.

And I did something real naughty. Boy, I can never forget that. See, our teacher get his hair long over this side. Because he's bald, so he leave his hair grow long. And he comb over, cover his bald head. And I notice that, because I wait long time, till he's fast asleep in the chair. And then all the kids waiting for action. And they know everybody like do that. He had a stick for pointer. I go up and grab the pointer. I lookin at everybody, they egg me on. So I put the pointer under the hair and I flip it over. Everybody bust out laughing. The whole class they laugh, laugh. Oh, my teacher woke up, you know. "Oh, Kakalina [Cathrine], you like fool, eh?" He joke and say that. He tell me, "You go on the blackboard 500 times, 'I must not fool in school.'" I gotta write five hundred time "I must not fool in school." Everybody went home already; only me in class. So I go write I, I, I, I…, Must, must, must… He erase 'em all. He tell me, "I must not fool in school." I gotta write all that 500 till after supper. But they kept my food when I came home. And never again I did that. Oh, teacher lookin like mad with me. Those guys they know I gutsy, yeah? I like play. Sometime I do that with the chair. I put water on the seat. And when they go to sit down, their clothes all wet. Hah, hah! And those guys they laugh. They wait for me make something likc that. But we get good fun.

So I go home and I get good scolding from Sarah. The girls go home first, yeah? They tell, "Sarah, Cathrine got punished. She gotta write on the board." "What she did?" "She put the teacher's hair on the other side." She said, "That's not good. It's wrong to do anything like that." But she was laughing. And then she said, "What you folks did?" "We laughed." She told, "You folks just as bad."

I was down there up to the fifth grade. And they had Edwin Lelepali [a young patient] just came in. Teacher tell him teach me how to read. But we only fight. I say, "You know how to read?" "Yeah." I say,"You read 'em then." We fight like that. That's why he hated me for the longest time. Now we all grown up, so we let it go that kind stuff.

Losing Sister Eunice

And when I went in, my sister Eunice, she was still there at Kalihi. So after, when I came out of the hospital, then they made me stay with her. And we fought all the time. You see, my sister… there was another girl that came in, and my sister was friendlier to her than me, you know, and I got upset. And she and I would just fight. And the following year, they asked her to go to Kalaupapa. But when my sister was sent, I cried. I cried. And all her clothes, I put 'em all in my bed when I slept, and I cried myself to sleep. Just like I loved the smell of her body, yeah? You know how kids are. It went on like that for weeks until Sarah told me, "You better throw those clothes away. They're dirty."

So they took her about 4:30 in the morning and her stuff. I went outside with my blanket. And my sister went on the truck. And I just cried. I was nine that time I think, nine or ten. And when the truck was loaded, I run after the truck and cry, "My sister, I like go too." They said, "You go home, you go home." But I still staying there and cry until they went out of the gate. And they closed the gate. And I just hung on that gate and I wen watch till I cannot see the truck no more. I look up the road, yeah? I can see the tail light and I knew she could see me. They close the canvas so the cars that follow cannot see them. Then they was stay down the pier and they go on the boat. About 8:00, then they start going on the ocean. They reach over here 3:00, afternoon.

And then came our turn. My sister left 1938 I think. And then 1942 we came. My sister died before I reached. She died the year before I came.

Attack on Pearl Harbor

I went in Kalihi 1937. I stayed there almost five years. The war broke out, I was fourteen years old. Yeah, I was well aware of the war, because we saw all the planes that came. They flew over us—oh, I would say just about a thousand feet above us. They came real low, just above the house. We was hiding under the eaves at the school. You see, it was Sunday morning, we was going to breakfast and all this commotion came up. That's when we start hearing the planes fly over. So many of them. And we say, "Gee, how come so much planes on Sunday?" We didn't know they're gonna attack Pearl Harbor. So we just watch the whole incident. Got a bird's eye view. We saw the whole thing before it happened. And then we saw the smoke, black smoke, cause they were bombing already. And we got scared. Cause we never thought anything like this could happen. We got scared and we wanted to hide. But we didn't have breakfast. When we came back again for lunch, a lotta the damage was done. A lotta people killed. We could hear the bombing. They was striking us from all over. They came from north shore side, and from the Diamond Head side.

But we stayed together at Kalihi for a few months, until they told us we are sending you up to Kalaupapa. Oh, we just cried our heart out. We didn't wanta leave Kalihi. They said it could be dangerous for us. Cause we were right in the danger zone [during World War Two]. They said that they would have to answer to our parents. Parents would say, "Why didn't you send them somewhere else?" Some of the kids stayed back because their parents said no.

Going to Kalaupapa

We all came up '42, same time. There were other girls that came up and stayed with their sister or their aunty. They cannot stay by themself. They outlaw that. I had a sister here, but she died before I reached. I didn't get to see her before she died. I'm glad in a way I didn't. Because she would have me stay with her. But I don't want that. I would rather live with the girls [at Bishop Home], yeah? We'd grown up together, all of us.

So they told us only one suitcase, no more than that. Ohhh, we have to leave a lot of things back, things we had. We had our lamps, our lampshade, a lotta pictures, our new glasses. And, you know, when we left, the other girls they stayed there, they all rushed up and helped themselves. They took all our things. And we thought that was so unfair. The Board of Health should have bought it from us. They gave only $25 each.

They ship us just like animals. We gotta be ready by 4:00 in the morning. And they have this big truck. We all sit on the seat, and they put a big canvas to hide us. You know, when you on the road, the cars stop in the back, yeah? And they can look inside. So they had a big canvas, heavy canvas, to protect us from being seen by the back cars. Then they drop us down the pier, way away from every peering eyes. Nobody on that side. Just the boat waiting for us, that's the S.S. Hawaii. We was all waiting for our loved ones to come say goodbye.

Lot of them came. They hug, kiss their loved one, then they go on the boat. I waited till the last, and I think my father could see me, but he never come. I don't know, I have feelings about my father. I think he was down there early, but I think my father was afraid of the disease. I think he was hiding someplace. He didn't want to come where I was. When we got on the boat, we was going out already, too far for stop or anything, then I saw my father. I loved him. When I say, "Papa, Papa," he waved at me. I don't know, he might be crying. I stayed there until I couldn't see.

It was nice, smooth all the way until we hit the channel, started to get rough. And when we went out in the deep water, we all got sick. I got dizzy. You know, when I get seasick I get dizzy. And I start running to the side of the boat.

And you know where they put us? Where the cattles are standing. We couldn't go downstairs. Put all the mattress on top and we gotta sit, and there're thirty-nine of us. And they had a big canvas to protect us from the sun and rain. That day it rained. It poured when we was in the channel. And the cow doodoo all over the place, and we had to stay with that smell till we reach. Not one of them would come down and shoot it with a hose. And we looked good those days. Maybe we never had eyebrows, eyelashes, but our face was perfect. But they were scared. And above us there's a railing like, and all the passengers came out to take a look at us. You know how we felt, to be stared at? They figure, well, they're only small kids, it doesn't matter. You know? But we are people; we need our privacy. We stayed like that till we reach. And guess what we had for toilet? Two cracker can. One was for the boys, one was for the girls. And there was only a canvas in the middle to separate us. Every time when you go toilet we had to take another girl with us, cause we don't know who's watching, or peeping. We were treated like part of the cattle.

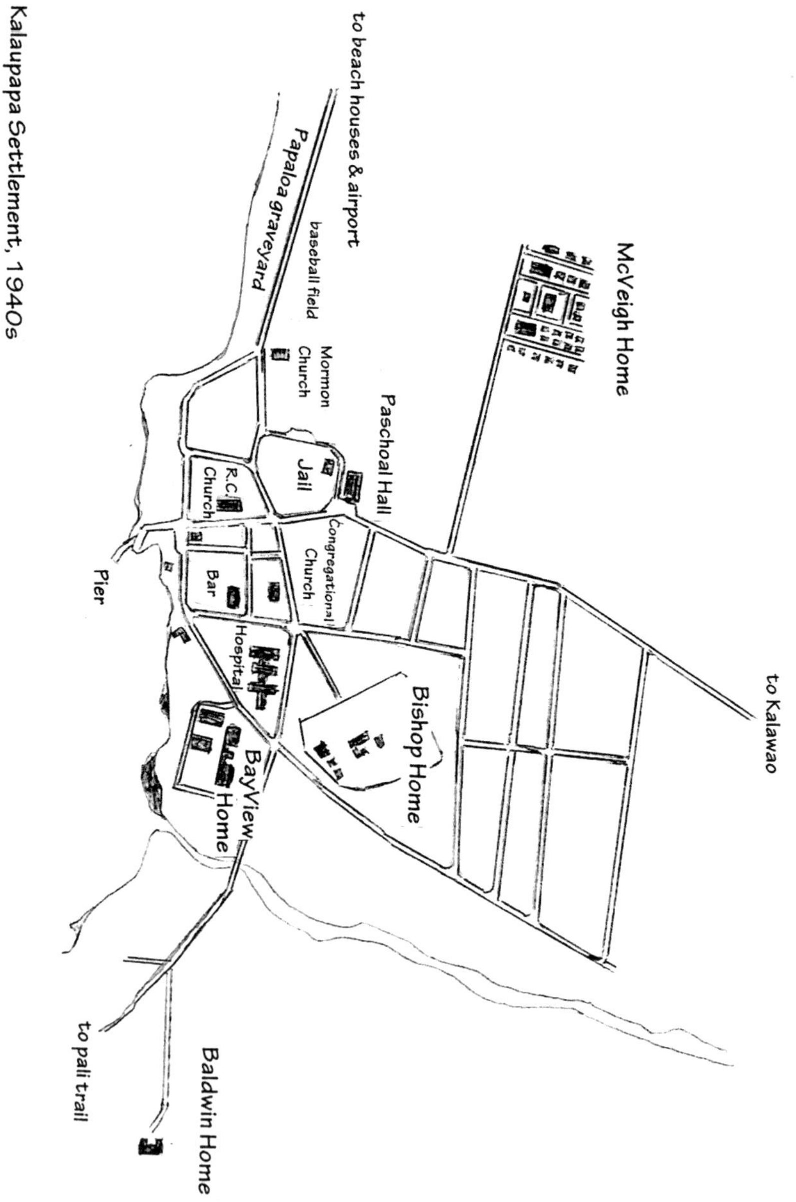
Kalaupapa Settlement, 1940s
to beach houses & airport
Papaloa graveyard
baseball field
McVeigh Home
Mormon Church
Paschoal Hall
Jail
R.C. Church
Congregational Church
Pier
Bar
Hospital
Bishop Home
BayView Home
to Kalawao
to pali trail
Baldwin Home

Chapter 2. A Teenager at Kalaupapa (1942 to 1947)

By the time we reach Kalaupapa, oh, the people. Was close to three hundred, maybe three hundred and fifty or more. All the sea wall was covered with people standing up. They all knew who was coming—the kids. The first time they going get kids in the settlement.

You know how grownups feel about kids, specially with this disease, yeah? The grownups they don't like kids, because kids stare and kids ask questions. But when we came out, Sarah briefed us up. She call us together, she say, "You know when you folks go out there Kalaupapa, don't stare at them. Don't ask them questions." She kept pounding us every time, you know? Telling us not to ask question, not to stare. She just wanted us to realize that it's something they don't like, the patients. They hate to be ask, "How come you like that?" They don't wanta answer that kind silly question. They get mad. And I know how they feel, because I don't like people ask me that too.

So when we got up here [to Kalaupapa], they had a motor launch sent out for us. The boat came out to pick us up. The boys say, "Let the girls go first." We say, "No, you should go first." "No, let the girls go first." So the girls came up, had about fifteen of us. And they was taking us, the boat started and they say, "All the old men are waiting for you folks." They like tease us. We got mad, we said, "Okay." We go up first, nobody came like that to us. But when the boys went up, lot of them had uncles. They say, "I got nephew over here," and they all come down for them. We laughing. Over here, some of us had mothers. Some had uncles, or aunties. And get plenty fathers.

First Days at Kalaupapa

And we got on shore. We all stood on shore, and we all look out at the people. I had two brothers. I was trying to look for my brother. I couldn't find them, because the two of them never go down to see me. They never like me back out from them like some do, yeah? They go up and they look at us, then they start backing away. They never like I do that to them. And I keep asking people, "Where's my brother Ah Wah?" "Oh, he's up the Baldwin Home." "Where's my brother Ah Chong [Samson]." "He's at the Baldwin Home." I didn't see them for days. I gotta ask somebody how I can go up there. So they brought me to Mother Marianne's grave and they say, "You see the road? Go straight down here. You keep goin all the way till you see a big boulder on the road. That's where your brother live." So I went by myself. And I saw somebody in the yard, I said, "Can I speak to Ah Wah? He's my brother." And they know I was new patient from Honolulu. Then they call my brother. He saw me, he back out, you know. He never like come. I run, I chase him. When I saw him, I said, "Hello, Ah Wah." He scratch his head. We embrace. And I cry. We both cry. And I tell I like see my brother Ah Chong [Samson]. My brother Ah Chong has tube in his throat cause he couldn't breathe. So I went to see him. He never like look at me. He was shame. I went up to him, I grab him, and then the three of us hugged. And we talked.

They shame cause they were disfigured. Just like I would be shame, if my family came that never see me for a long time. You change, you know. You look good one time, the next time you changing. Your muscles give up. You get paralysis. Your eyes don't work good. We always rubbing our eyes. They just fill up with water. And then the skin gets loose. And then the duct get swelled up because it sags and your eye get dry. They tell you you come blind if you going do that. When I came I was in good shape. It's too bad—somebody took my picture but I don't have it anymore. I was cute. I had a beautiful nose. Yeah, that was the only picture I had that I look good. And people we knew from Kalihi looked so different. A lot of people died. Some of the girls that they were at Kalihi, they were so attractive. So when I came up, I went looking for one girl, her name was Mary Anne, attractive Hawaiian girl. She sort of took me under her wing after my sister left Kalihi. She was good to me. You see those days, there're a lotta girls drinking, and carousing with men, yeah? A lotta men, they just fool around the girls and one guy took over three, four wahines. But she was full of vitality and energy, and so pretty. But I saw her at the end. I walked to the hospital at Kalaupapa, I say, "I want to see Mary Anne," cause they tell me where she was. When I talked to her, I look at her face. Ohhh, it wasn't her at all. She had no eyebrow, no eye-lashes. Her lips was covered with dressing. You know, they were raw, yeah? I said, "Mary Anne?" Say "Yeah it's me." I went to her and I hugged her. And I cried. She said, "Don't cry." I don't know what she had, but she didn't live long.

But we disappointed cause the [government] store, they don't sell candy or ice cream, they only sell grocery. We run in the store. "I like ice cream." "Oh, no more." "I like candy." "No more." Oh my, we look so sad. Then we found other store. It was run by Jonah M. He had ice cream, candy, crackerjack, cookies—all what we like. We just sat there and ate all we like. And there was other stores down at Papaloa, they sell crack seed and soda, beer. They even had chop suey house, saimin house. See there were a lot of people. It was worthwhile having a store. Not today. The store Gloria run [now],[4] all they sell is beer, wine, ice cream, maybe seeds, candy. That's enough.

And they open a school for us. Because there're two teachers had the disease. There was Cecilia A. from Honolulu, she was a former teacher. And Ada L. from Hawai'i Island.

---

[4] At the time of this story, there was a store run by the state and another private store in Kalaupapa, called Fuesaina's and run by patient Gloria Marks.

Life at Bishop Home with Sarah[5]

Sarah was at Kalihi Hospital and she was taking care of herself. And then, when the girls kept coming in, one after another, and they look at our age, it's too young, we need somebody to help us. Then they called Sarah up at the office. They told Sarah if she could be a mother to us, teach us all about womanhood, you know. She said, "I'll try." Sarah was about twenty-four that time. [After that] Sarah was taking care of us. And she taught us all about how to become a woman. We needed a woman to tell us—how to cook, how to sew, bake. She did a lot for us.

Bishop Home was a nice place to live, only ladies. The younger girls stayed one side, and the older ones stayed down. Some of them was very upset when we came. They had to move out. The nuns told them, "You folks have to move down the other side, cause these girls are coming are all underage and they need a place to be together." So one of them didn't wanta move, she said, "I'm not moving. I'm gonna stay here." And they say, "Alright." We drove her nuts. She took off. We were always yelling around. Poor thing. And we always niele [ask curious questions] and all this. She got tired of us. So we helped her move. She went down the other side.

Sarah even taught us how to kill chicken. This stray chicken came into Bishop Home. (They told us any cat, dog, chicken that strayed in we could keep.) He was a rooster. We called him Chickadee. He followed us around everywhere. And then we taught him to stay home, so he don't make doodoo on the porch. Then one day Sarah told us take him behind and kill him. So we go back there and we're passing the knife back and forth. "You do it." "Oh no, you do it." Pretty soon we hear Sarah say, "You killed him yet?" Finally she came back, said, "Give me the knife." And she killed him. Then she made us clean him

[5] Sarah came with the girls when they came to Kalaupapa in 1942 and they all lived at Bishop Home.

and she cooked him. And somebody else had given us another chicken, so she cook 'em both. And when we asked, "Which one is Chickadee?" she said, "That one." So we all ate the other one. Then afterward, she told us was Chickadee we ate. Ohhhh.

And Sarah, all the men were chasing for her. Sarah was very attractive when she came up here. And the men were after her, you know. A lot of them were Filipinos. Used to write letters, and mail 'em in the post office. She look at it, she get upset. She tell, "Oh, another one." So she give us the letter, we read the letter. It say, "Oh, my heart is broken for you. I in love with you." All that kind silly stuff. And she get angry, you know. Until she found the one she love. That was far after. Sarah came out here she was thirty-two. I think she was thirty-six she got married.

When we came up here, we came up as a group, and we always worship together. Every afternoon about 6:00 Sarah used to have us do 'ohana [family religious service]. She call us in. Somebody yell, "'Ohana." Then the word pass on to all the girls. We leave our bicycle, whatever we was playin with, we take off home. We had our 'ohana—Catholic, Protestant, Mormon—all together. Sarah taught us how to pray. We sing a song, have evening prayer, sing again, say twenty-third psalm, sing again, do closing prayer, "Our Father." If we had fought or done wrong, that's the time we ask for forgiveness.

We just stayed together so we didn't think that we needed to go separately to Catholic church, Mormon church. I think was either the second or the third Sunday, Sarah talked to us. When came Sunday, the girls all got dressed, and they was all headed the same way, to the Protestant church. Sarah said, "No, you have to go to your own church." Said, "You, you, you, you, you're all Catholic. You go to the Catholic." Oh, they start crying, say, "We don't wanta go Catholic church. We wanta go with you folks." Cause Sarah is Protestant, I was lucky. Because I was Protestant, I got to stay with Sarah. But the other girls, they had to go. Sarah said, "You go to your own church. I don't wanta hear anything more." Was hard to part. Sarah said, "We'll see you at lunch. When you pau [finished with] church, you come home." Just the breaking away was…for young kids it's hard. Cannot accept it. They cried, you know. And the Mormon girls went to their own church, they was not happy at all. We were happy because we were Protestant and we got to stay with her. There was about six of us I think. The whole row was taken by us. Yeah, that was a terrible time we went through, when Sarah had to tell us where we gotta go, what we gotta do. It's just like part of growing up, yeah? We just didn't want the separation. But Sarah say, "I cannot let you folks do that. Because they going think I'm holding you folks back. I'm not." I don't know if somebody went to see Sarah. Probably the nuns talked to Sarah. "I understand you have some girls Catholic. We want them to come to the Catholic church." So that's how Sarah got on the ball, I guess.

Then the Catholic church was having a procession up to Bishop Home and we all wanted to be in it. It was a celebrating day for some saint or something. Corpus Christi I think. And we were all young girls. And they told us, "You folks have to wear all white, carry a basket with flower petals, and when you walk from the church, you start throwing petals." "Oh yeah, we like do that." Cause we were young children. And then the grownup wen stick their noses inside. That made us angry. Cause we couldn't do it. Because somebody went to see somebody down the Catholic church, said our girls are not coming. And the Mormon girls are not coming. So only had the Catholic girls. There were about five of them. And we were dressed all in white, we still had our basket flowers, we were crying in church. I look at my minister, I hated her for stopping us. So then we can hear the music, and then singing. Then our minister was talking, we was trying to look outside the window. Oh, we stay crying and crying. Then Reverend Alice talk to us. She said, "Children, you must understand that when there's something like this going on, and you have your church, your church comes first. That's why we didn't want you folks to join them, because we have Sunday service, and this is where you supposed to be, in your own church." Oh, was hard for us to take. And then we can hear all the music, they singing, and you know the girls throwing. They went up to Bishop Home, they went around Bishop Home, they stop at the chapel little while.[6] And then they continue on down and they went around the Catholic church. We can hear them singing. Oh, was a sad day for us. We went home from church, nobody like talk. We stubborn.

You know, when we first came up here, we thought we were all gonna live together and we all have our meals together. And we found out that only the girls over here at Bishop Home. And the boys are down the other side at Baldwin Home. And some boys, and some girls, went up the other side to McVeigh Home. And we feel sorry about that, you know. We miss being together. We were brought up like brothers and sisters at Kalihi. We all ate together. We all played together. But this time, no, they were away from us. And we got kinda lonesome, we missed them. And when we see them the next day, "What you folks had for lunch?" "Oh, we had this." "What you folks had for supper?" "Oh we had that." We just like know what they had. And they ask us, I always tell that we had the best dining room in the settlement. "How come?" "Well, we get tablecloth, and we had plates, knife, spoon, teaspoon, cup and saucer, glass, napkin." They say, "All that?" "Yeah, just like haole." "Oh, yeah? Well you guys lucky. Us we just throw one bowl and one spoon." "That's all you guys get?" Because we like compare, yeah? "Never get a cup?" "No. Only the fork get sometime." Oh, we had the best dining room. The nuns were so good to us. Then came Christmas, they'll give us the napkins they get flowers. We gotta color all the flowers. We had color crayons, and we color the four color, and then when you got through you can make a decoration with your napkin. And put on the plate, folded-up-like napkin. And you know the table looks so nice. They bring out white

[6] Bishop Home has its own little Roman Catholic chapel, St. Elizabeth's, in addition to the main Roman Catholic church in Kalaupapa Settlement, St. Francis.

table cloth. Beautiful. In the center we had poinsettias. Oh, my goodness, look so nice. So we loved it at Bishop Home.

The nuns were good cooks. The head of the cook was Sister Margaret. Sister Margaret was just like the kind chef. And had Sister Anne, she was the second in command. And then we had Sister Mary Anne. And some did the pastry, some did something else, salads maybe. And Sister Margaret would make beef roast. Sister made that, oh we like that. And she make pipikaula [dried beef strips] for us. She make 'em dry. She hang a long wire along the stove. They got the kind big burner, yeah? And she clean all the meat, hanging down, all along the wire while the stove is hot. It dries the meat. And we know next day we going get pipikaula. Ooh. The nuns fry the onion, pipikaula, tomato—all cut up—poi. And then another day, on Kuhio Day, all the kind. Hawaiian kind [food], yeah?

So I worked at the kitchen. And you know what? Used to get dollar one day. For us it's big pile money, dollar one day. Before, they used to pay us all in silver dollars, not paper money. They give us one package, it's thirty or thirty-one silver dollars. We didn't know the value of the silver dollars, but all the businessmen, they were outside waiting for us. "You like change? you like change?" "Yeah, yeah, too heavy." Hoh, they quick time they give us thirty-one dollars or thirty dollars, yeah? according to what we have. They get big smile on their face.

For lü'au, they ask us to make cakes. We make four chocolate cake, four prune cake, four coconut cake, and four cream cake. And they paid for all that. So Sarah keeps our kitty. And end of the year, she tell us how much we had. And if we like make a dinner, we can buy. So that's how we do. End of the year, we celebrate for all our hard work make cake.

And when we live in Bishop Home, every Monday, Wednesday and Friday get movie up at the [Paschoal] Hall. But we had English movies Monday and Friday. And on Wednesday we get either Japanee or Filipino movie, because they are the other ethnic groups here. And they like to see their kind movie, yeah? We all go. We didn't understand what they saying. We all go. And the girls would hang out in the yard, picking all the flowers, and we make the kind flower with the fern, you know on the side. But all our head just covered with flowers. We thought that was beautiful; it would catch the eye of the boys. They sit not too far from us. Ha, ha! So we figure they'll be looking at us. They had lotta flowers in Kalaupapa, lotta rose bushes all over the place. So we cut the rose, we add 'em to the ferns—maidenhair, all that kind. We loved that changeable rose, because sturdy. The other rose could fall off, the petal. So then, when we finish our lei for our head, we put it on the basin, we sprinkle water. The next girl put on the basin, sprinkle water. Next one. So that cover all the basin. Sarah comes, Sarah say, "Whose rose are this?" She like use the basin. All these leis got in the way. She got so mad, she put all our leis outside the porch. She said don't put it on the basin, because people like to use the basin. We think we look beautiful, ohhh. Well, you know when you young you think different, yeah? Now I think back, I think how silly. But we didn't realize. Aw, golly.

Swimming

Down this side, closer to the graveyard, there's a nice place to swim. The sharks so far never did come in there. Over there I almost got drowned. We just came up here, I think was less than a month we was here. So we asked Sarah, she could drive us, we wanta go swim. We didn't know how to swim. Lucky Sarah told us, "You folks cannot go until you folks take somebody older who can swim." So we went looking all over for somebody, and I found this girl Carrie. She's my family, you know, we related. And she said, "Okay, I can do that." Cause she family. So. It was low tide, I went out between two rocks, I stood on one. It was over here for me {chest high]. And then, I felt like a big fish bumped my leg and I went off the rock. Oh, over my head. Was deep. I came up, I start yelling, "Help! Help! Help!" I go down again, I come up. "Help! Help!" Screaming, Carrie heard me screaming, but she thought I was joking. She said, "You really want me to save you?" I tell, "Yeah." She jumped in the water. She a good swimmer. She was big, you know. She come, she talk to me first, she said, "I let you on my back, but don't pull me under." She say, "Relax. Kinda float." "Yeah, okay." "Don't pull me under now. Otherwise you and I going drown." So I just let myself go up. And she swam me in, take me on her back. Oh, but I had good scolding from Sarah. She say, "Why did you go out there? You should have stayed inshore where you can stand up." I didn't know it was that deep because I was standing on the rock. But when I fell off the rock, oh my goodness. It was over six feet deep. So I got back safe. Never again I went out that far.

After that first incident Sarah said, "You guys learn how to swim." So we had to go down the pier, with somebody who know how to swim. But they taught us how to swim. Learn how to float on our back. And if you can do that, you can learn how to swim. So all of us was in the water, learn how to float. It don't seem that hard. We stayed on our backs long time. So now she said, "Try get up and swim." At first we had hard time. We swim like a dog, so it kept us afloat. Then she started to swim, and she tell us to follow her. So just like that we learn how to swim. Down by the pier.

But those days we had so much fun swimming. And we wouldn't swim when it's really rough. The waves used to be about fifteen feet high right in the pier. So the boys would tie a big rope from one end to the other end. And they always tell us to hold the rope when the wave coming. So it won't dash us against something. So we see the wave coming, big wave, and we grab on the rope. And we hang. Everybody was screaming and laughing. And we had so much fun. Those days are really gone forever, because everybody got old. The most of them died. And nobody came down there to scold us, but we shouldn't be swimming that kind time, cause it's dangerous. But when you're young, you get more guts than brains, yeah? And then when you get older, you wanta tell the next young person to watch out. You're different now, you're not as brave as you used to be.

And people used to come to the pavilion, down by the pier. And they would just sit there and watch us. Because when they were young, I think they do the same thing. But now they all grown up, and it's not fun anymore. They cannot go in the water cause they had sore feet and the doctor don't want them breaking their feet. Or they had sore hands. And sometimes they have the boat running around, and they come in and pick us up if you wanted to go ride.

Sometime the whales would come and they would swim around and then spout. Mother and one baby. They just trying to show him around, yeah? And then never take long, then the dolphins come. And everybody say, "Gee, we are so fortunate to be at the right place, where you can watch the show for free." The dolphins would just go dive, up, and around, you know? They were so fast. You see, the sharks are scared of the dolphins. The dolphins go in schools, and the sharks they go either one or two. So they are afraid of the dolphins, because they charge. And by the time they get through with the shark, the shark gets all banged up. They poke 'em with their nose and then the shark turn around and leave.

The Kalaupapa Itch

You were not a citizen until you get the itch, you know? Everybody comes here they pick up the Kalaupapa Itch. And then we go see the doctor and the doctor prescribe this Danish ointment.[7] This Danish ointment is made from yellow [boric] ointment and that acid stuff [sulphur]. It's yellow, powdery. One day we went to see the doctor and we was worried about what we had. We had blisters all

[7] It is not clear what caused this "Kalaupapa Itch." Danish ointment is a polysulfide preparation used to treat various skin disorders that result from Demodex mites (David Tse, Demodex Treatment, abst-48-Demodex-Treatment - HairSite.com).

over our bodies. You know, lumps, and water would come out and leave a little hole. He look at us, he smile. He said, "All of you have it?" And we said, "Yeah!" He said, "OK, you be my guest." He put us all in the hospital and he put us on a liquid diet for three darn days. We had crackers and soup, fruit and juice, and tea, and that's all we had. It was like this for three days. And you know, he made the nurse rub that terrible smell all over our body. It's just like car grease. That's what it looks like, and it stinks. They rub it all over our body, and when you get through, we walk just like zombies. We don't wanna stay one place, we keep walking around. Until in the evening when you start to dry up on your body, and the clothes don't feel that sticky, so we jump in the bed and cover ourself up. And we close the side door because the boys wanna come and tease us, you know? They call us wa'owao. Wa'owao is itch. They say, "Eh, wa'owao!" We nevah like them tease us that, you know. We had to stay in the hospital three days with that stink medicine and even the diet was for three days. The third day the nurses put us in the shower and they bathe us and the girls help each other scrub the back you know? Finally, we all out of there. And when we all go through with that, the doctor said, "OK, girls. You wanna go home now or this evening?" We all said, "Now! We wanna get outta here!" And we all took off. And Dr. Sloane he told us, "Now, you are Kalaupapa citizens. You have to have the itch." We went home to Bishop Home and the boys tease us. We said, "You folks going get 'em, too. You wait." And they all got it. And when the boys had to go inside, we took a walk in the evening and we yell, "Wa'owao! wa'owao!" And they turn away from us. Yeah, you have to have that. Everybody gotta have the Kalaupapa Itch.

You see, you know how we got it? Through the linen, the laundry. They wash our clothes in the funny kine soap, you know? And then they add this stuff inside, just like for the dogs. But it was affecting us, you know? So after we found out that it was the linen, we did our own washing. Aunty Sarah told us, "We do our own laundry from now on." So that's what we did.

Schooldays (1942-45)

When I came to Kalaupapa, I went back fifth grade. I wasn't that smart. The only thing I was good in was hygiene, geography, and spelling. The worst one I hated was arithmetic. Ohhh. I watch the person next to me writing so I could copy. Then teacher tell me, "How did you get this?" "I don't know." Hah, hah! Oh, I tell you. When I was in school Kalihi I do that. I did the same kolohe [naughty] stuff in here. And we had two teachers, Cecilia A. and Ada L. Was me, Winifred, and plenty other kids. And Winifred, we made her cry one time. They told her what was this word. "Deter-mine". Everybody laugh. Supposed to be determine, but she say "deter-mine." And the kids always tease each other. Then when I got mine, they laugh at me. "How you got this?" "I don't know." (laughs) I was not good at arithmetic.

And then I wrote something on a paper one day and I pass 'em to all the kids. They laugh, they giggle. Cecilia A. say, "May I have that paper?" So I look at them, ohhh. I wrote on top, "We the children of Kalawao School wish to have Ada L's body on view in the Bishop Museum." That's the other teacher up here. She laughed, she never scold me, you know. I think I going make one more note, I going use her name. So I make one more note, I put Cecilia A. "We the children of Kalawao County, we like to have Cecilia A. body on view in Bishop Museum." And it went around again. And she saw it. She said, "What do you have there? Let me have that." Ooh! I think, oh no. She read it, she start crying. The tears came down her eyes. I think, "Gee, what wrong I did now?" Because with the other schoolteacher she laugh; I put her name, now she cry. So I don't know what wrong I did. Then she took the note home to the husband. Her husband John, he likes me, treat me like a daughter, He call me up the house. He said, "Cathrine, you're a naughty girl. Why did you do this?" So I look at the note, I say, "Oh I never do nothing wrong." He said, "You didn't write it? Look at this." I said, "I write the same note. I use Ada L's name. Your wife laugh." He said, "What?" "Your wife laughed when I put Ada L's name. But when I put her name, she got mad." He went in there, he said, "Cecilia, you come out here." He went go for her, he tell, "Why didn't you stop that when she did the first one. You was wrong to laugh at it. She thought it was funny, so she use your name then." She had a good scolding by her husband. I look at them, I scared already. I take off, I go home. Yeah. I troublemaker in school, you know. The school was dull, that's why. No action. Nobody like do anything. Nobody gutsy enough to do something kolohe. So I did it

So when came summer vacation, the state put us on the sampan--only the girls would go—put us on the sampan and they would take us back to Honolulu for summer vacation. One month, Kalihi Hospital. And then when we come back the boys would go for one month. And then by the time they come back, ready for school. The boat too small for both. Cause there was a lot of us, and the captain don't want too much. Too heavy yeah? We would have loved that the boys go, so we can fight on the boat, you know? No, but they went after us.

I would call Auntie Kapeka. I tell, "Auntie. I'm home here at Kalihi." "Oh. How come you came down here?" Auntie is that kind, yeah? She don't wanta make anything wrong. I tell, "No, they bring us down for the school vacation. And then we going back again." Then she start crying, and crying. She come down and see me. All the whole battalion come down to see me. She look at me, she say, "Oh, you getting worse." I don't know, maybe to them, yeah? But I felt the same. My face was still, yet, unchanged. But she saw some changes in me.

We only go up to eighth grade at Kalaupapa, yeah? I was eighteen, you know, and you no finish eighth grade eighteen, eh? High school you finish eighteen. But was only intermediate. They had to get rid of us. Had about four of us was eighteen. So, we had commencement in the big hall [Paschoal Hall]. Mrs. A made a nice commencement for us. We march in, she play the piano. And you know the song that go, da, da, da, dah, dee, dee, dee, dee, dee? It's a march like. We learn how to sing that song, and we dress all in white. For the boys, white shirt with black pants. We march in, oh, everybody clap for us. And we stand up all in line. And we had recital, we had to say something. And everybody was call up for their diploma. And then everybody clap. And after the commencement, had plenty people had leis for us. They went ahead and make plumeria lei, and orchid leis for us. And that was the last. We never had school at Kalaupapa after that. Because Mister Judd [the Kalaupapa Administrator] thought it was wise to send all those who like get ahead, go down Hale Mohalu [in Pearl City] and go for high school.[8] So lot of the girls did. They took up the challenge and they went for high school. And we missed them.

Tutu Hukia

Oh, my grandfather Hukia go for ʻöhua [baby manini fish]. He lived right down by the beach. And he told me if I like see that kind, I come early morning. So I came down about 5:00 in the morning from Bishop Home. And then he was going to go catch ʻem. Yeah, it's transparent. He said because the sun no come up yet, it's still early in the morning. And he caught it right in front of his house. Get plenty rocks, you know, but he just throw the net over. And I say, oh this kind, no more bone. And he tell, yeah. And he stick ʻem in his mouth right over there. Oh the tail going like that, you know. Oh my. I tell, "No make, no make [not dead yet]." It was still yet alive. He say "Oh, ʻono,ʻono [delicious]."

Hukia, that was his name. I call him Tūtū Hukia. He sort of hänai [adopt] me. Because I was walking by myself down over by the beach. And these two [the man and his wife] was sitting down in their

[8] Hale Mohalu was a facility for Hansensʻs disease patients in Honolulu, mostly for patients with less advanced cases of the disease. Settlement Administrator Lawrence Judd (1947-49) established a high school program there for the young patients at Hale Mohalu and also offered those at Kalaupapa a chance to attend.

old garage they turn into a sitting room. They had a house close to the beach. But they had a old garage that they didn't use for car anymore. They sort of fix it up with mattress and lauhala [pandanus] mats, like a place to rest. And they left the door open, and they could see the water. But every afternoon they went down there. Cause sometime hot, yeah? And that's a nice place cool off. Just sit down there and look out to the ocean.

And the husband would go down throw net for fish in front. The old lady say, ahh, she think maybe he have good luck. So I stick around, he throw. Oh, he had küpïpï and all kind different fish. He brings 'em up and he clean 'em. He cut 'em all up and make raw. For her, his wife. I call her Tūtū Lady. They adopted me. They saw me walking by myself, and she say I look like her grand-daughter, so she called me. I went up there and I sat down. And we start talking, and she told me if I like I can come next week. They was lonely. But like I was what they was waiting for, one kid to come along and be with them. So I went there every Sunday. And he went down to the beach every Sunday, he caught something and he make raw, with the limu [seaweed], 'inamona [kukui nut relish], and we all ate together. And when we rode the car I sat in the middle and the grandmother on the side, and they thought like I was theirs, you know. And I really felt good, because I left my grandmother and my grandfather home. They sort of took their place. So I felt good, I never felt like my grandmother and grandfather was lost, like they was with me.

Sometime he would go down and make some 'opihi [limpet]. Cause his legs were good, he could go in the water. His hand were good, just maybe two fingers missing, yeah? But he could do a lot in the water. Always like to throw-net. And then they get papio, this kind size. And they know the seasons [for] throw-net they catch the papio. And you could see the silver in the water, this big smile on his face. You know sometime these old people are clever. Sometime they throw something in the water. I just think it's water, but I think it's kinda numb the fish around there. And then they don't swim very fast, then they get groggy. I think they had ‘awa root in their yard to use. They chew ‘em and they stick inside.

I love the manini. They have the white meat and they look like a very clean fish. All they eat is limu, you know. So she taught me how to eat it with the guts. Oh, all I taste was bitter. It tastes bitter, but it’s that kind of limu they eat. They get pū pa‘akai [sharing of salt], with the salt in the mouth, and take away that bitter taste.

They make their own poi, and put the meat inside when they eat the poi. He had a taro patch. Not too far from the Mormon Church he had a big patch. He took me behind there. That’s where he mend his net. He had house, he had a lotta net in there. When he go out there, clean the taro patch, I go in the taro patch with him too. Clean all that kind stuff growing inside. And they let the pipe go to the taro patch from the person who lives right next door. He had the water running all the time. And he pull taro, and then he bring ‘em back to the house. And then they would cook the taro, peel the taro, and he’d pound. He had the pounder and the board, yeah? So he would pound. And I would look at him, I said, ohhh, just like my grandfather.

He loved me. He really loved me. I had a nodule in my eye [from Hansen’s disease]. When his wife didn’t wanta give me the medicine for my eye, he was angry with her. She thought I was too young. She used to say, “One time you miss, no good.” You have to continue like antibiotics, gotta keep on, yeah? So one time you miss, it throws everything off. So he tell her, “Never mind. She going do ‘em. She going do ‘em.” He look at me, he tell me, “Baby, you follow what Tutu lady tell you.” “Yeah, okay.” “There, you see? she going do ‘em.” And then she gave me the medicine. It was the pöpolo leaf. You see, some they’re very particular. They say three leaves, six leaves, that’s what you have to follow. You pick it up before the sun go down. So I was kinda curious, you know, why? She said because after the sun go down, all kind pïlau [bad] spirits all around. And that’s true. That’s when they come out and take you, the kölohe [wicked] things, yeah? And they try block the medicine from helping you. So I listen. Before the sun go down I pick ‘em up already. You put it with your own saliva, chewing the pöpolo leaf, that’s how you make the medicine.

But there’re two kinds pöpolo, the one with purple flower and one with white flower. That’s the one you use, the white. Purity, yeah? The other, the seeds are good to eat, you can eat the seeds. But the white one is the medicine. See, the old folks, they know plenty, but they so scared to give ‘em out. Cause some people, they think we take three nights, but we’re not, some you have to go seven or four, some five, but mine was twenty-five. See, she just said twenty-five. So you gotta chew that and let somebody help put for me, cause I cannot. Ooh, it burns, just like alcohol. She said, “You go sleep. No eat, no stay up, go sleep.” The next day I get up, I get hard time open my eye. Just like pipili [glue], yeah? I had to pry it open. And then I wash all the piapia [matter], all that stuff that’s inside, coming out little by little. And I look at my eye, it was just like all red, you know. But when I do that for twenty-five days, and then I look in the mirror, no more the lump. Gone. So I went down to see her, tell, “Tutu, look.” I show her my eye, she say, “Ahh.” But she know already.

That’s why when the Hawaiians try teach you, you have to listen. Because it’s hard for them give away secrets like that if you’re not going listen. Pohö [useless]. You know, it’s a waste of time. But when you listen, it helps you, you lucky. This other girl that stayed with me in the same room, I tried to tell her to use that. She never believe that it could help. The doctor cauterized her eye. Ohhh, boy. She had a big scar on her eye for life. She gotta use her finger to put in the bowl water [during the cauterization]. If she takes it out, she going get shock. But how can you… somebody gotta hold you hand. You going get so scared from that thing, you going lift you hand out, you know. Oh, she was sick for days. She was in terrible pain afterward. So I tell her, “See, I told you try the Hawaiian medicine.” You see, she’s a pretty girl. But she got scar on her eye.

Camping (1944-46)

You know the picnic ground [at Judd Park at Kalawao]? You cross over—there's a board go across to the other side—that's where our camp was. It used to be the girl scout and boy scout camp. It's down by the beach, right on the cliff. From there you can see right inside Waikolu Valley and up Wailei'ia Valley. (See Map 1 in the Appendix.) It's outside, before Wailei'ia. It used to be real nice, only grass. But after we pau [finish] go camp, they never kept up.

We used to take up one, two, three, four tents. The first tent was for the sheriff and his dog. They have to chaperone us. We're all young girls, yeah? And then the Sisters, the nuns, said, "We want you folks to take care of our girls." So the sheriff had to go up with us. He stayed all night with us, with his own tent. And next to him we have two scoutmasters, they were patient. So they stayed in the next tent. And then the other two tent had six girls in each tent, so twelve of us. So then we stayed there one month. Oh, we loved it, we had a grand time. Every day different girls go cook. They think up the menu and they cook breakfast, lunch, supper. And then, next day two other girls cook breakfast, lunch, supper. We thought it was fun, every girl take turn cook. And every day was something different. And the two girls are the boss of the kitchen for that day. And there was a cat that it always came when we had our meal. So we left one day, and we saw him looking at us, you know. So we said, "Why don't we take the cat home? Cause he's going come back, look for us." He was tame already. So we pick him up, took him on the truck with us. We held him, and he never struggle. Said we're gonna call him Kalawao. And we keep him, and he was our cat. He stay with us until he died.

And every day it was the same thing. The sheriff got up early, start the fire for us, yeah? Start the fire, make the hot water. So when we get up, we come inside and he say, "Oh, I get the hot water going." "Oh, okay." Then,"What you girls going cook?" "Oh. Gonna make scrambled eggs, with the vienna sausage." Then he help us open the can. So we make all up. We mix 'em up, throw 'em in the fry pan. He help us. Then we put all the food on the table—cracker, eggs, toast—and all the dishes that you need. Then you go out there, you get triangle, yeah? Ba-dang! ba-dang! ba-dang! All the girls get up, they start coming. Was so much fun.

But that was just for that time. Now we all old. All we have is memories. And you know, Lucy and I are the only ones to remember. When we had off time, we could go swimming, we could go fishing, we had the time to play. And then we always had to watch the time. The two girls going cook had to leave early. The rest could stay till 11:00. And we went up, we start thinking of what we going cook. "What we going cook for lunch?" "Fried spam and eggs." "Oh, nice." "Tomato and lettuce, with mayonnaise." You know, we talk about it. "We said, okay, that'll be good." So we fry the spam, and egg, and then we have fried potato. And for vegetable--you gotta get vegetable—tomato and lettuce, or cucumber. We just throw everything together. And we feed the driver of the truck and we feed the helper. The helper was Henry Nalai'elua. They pick up our groceries and take it up to us. So, when get grocery day, everybody is in there, we check what we ordered from the store at Kalaupapa. And those days we get $10 each for ration. We check 'em all up. "Okay, we got everything." Then the girls start stashing 'em away in the closet. And then, that's when the girls start planning for some place to go, with all the girls that are going, eh? We make plan Thursday. Tell we going get up early, eat breakfast, and we go inside Waikolu. So we pick up all the gingers, we make lei. Then we come home, we pick up the kīkania.[9] Those days had lotta kīkania, all over. Come Friday night, we all going come home [to Kalaupapa]. When we go to the movie we get plenty lei on our head, on our neck. You know we smell so good.

---

[9] *Kīkania (Solanum aculeatissimum)* is a native plant that bears round, scarlet fruits that are often strung into *lei*. The *lei* of *kīkania* is considered the traditional *lei* of Kalaupapa.

Tidal Wave (1946)

The tidal wave came April Fool's Day. They nevah know how severe it was [going to be]. They just thought high seas, cause had high sea every time. We was all home up at Bishop Home. But Helen was working at Bay View Home. She come running home, and tell us. She said, "Oh, tidal wave! Oh, the water came up, you know? The house going down. " I look at her and say, "April Fool!" She said, "No! No!" She start crying, crying. Then I look at her. "No, I don't lie," she said, "go look for yourself." We went down the pier. And then we saw what the water did. The water came way up. It turned the office building around. The office was facing the mountain, but the wave turn it facing Oahu. That's how strong the water was. Lucky nobody was around there, because it would have taken them out. You know we saw the pier, no more water. Quarter of a mile out, no more water. Even down the black sand, all dry. The water wen suck way out and you could see the rocks and where the deep place, you know? And we watch from up high. Oh my goodness! And you can see water coming back, you know? Coming back. Oh, wen fill up. Came right up to the warehouse. Oh, and then it came on the land. It didn't come as a wave, it just rise up, even with the cement.

The water must have been 50 to 100 feet high, coming from the Aleutian Islands. The big wave build up, build up, came to north of Kalaupapa. You know, it came over all the papa [beach-side flats], went on the airport. 'As how big the wave was, coming over. And then it took Spud's beach house out. See that beach house was the biggest beach house in Kalaupapa. It was a green house with big porch. We get luaus outside there and they had a huge kitchen facing to the ocean. And they had about three or four bedrooms, and we slept down there, we all pile up in one room. That were a house that belonged to Spud. He just thought, "I get up early. I going work." He wanted to start the boiler early. So he left his houseand he went down to the laundry. And

I think 7:00 it struck. That house was so huge. And they had so many cats living with them. I think the whole batch went out. They were all on the porch, the cats; they were on the roof top. We could see them. And then all we saw was the top of the house going down, down. It went down slowly, so for awhile I thought maybe shallow enough it going stay like that, you know. No, it went down until the roof cannot see. And nobody could go out and help them, because the wave was coming back again. Everybody was scared. Then the house just went under. And I guess the cats all drowned. I still can see the wave. I stay there long time just watching, watching. And then somebody call me, "Come on! We go! We had one, two, three, four, I think five beach house was washed away and one was knocked down. And they nevah go fix 'em cause they figure it might come again, yeah?

And it [the tidal wave] kept going for the graveyard, and it emptied all the water into the baseball park. Tons of water. The graveyard was destroyed because the cross was on the grave was all knock over, all push down to the road. Nobody knew where to put it cause some of us wasn't here that long. And then the oldtimers said, "I think was over here." So we try and put where it was.

But the biggest fun was me and Puanani. We was at Bishop Home, and she said, "Eh, we go down check." So I said, "Okay." She and I went down and we was on the road almost to the Mormon Church. We saw all this thing on the road, and was squid. That darn squid – got five of them. And had chicken on the road. All wet the feather and they were half dead, you know. So I tell her, "We pick up the squid and the chicken." You know I had good hand that time. So she hold three chicken, I hold three chicken. And then we get the squid, put 'em inside our dress, pile 'em all up, we run home. We never leave one squid back. They saw us. "Sarah! Look what they get." She said, "Squid! And chicken!" She said,"You guys go pull all the feather out and then put 'em all in the ice box so they stay fresh." So we did that.

Now we run down again. And then we went down the beach and

the water was going out. Had this big blue ‘uhu [parrotfish], big one. Look like the water went way up and then when it came back, look like he got stuck on the sand. He was jumping up and down. I look at that, I tell her, "‘Uhu!" She said, "You like I go get ‘em?" "Yeah." We look outside, the water going out yet. We run down the sand. And we couldn't hold ‘em cause slippery. You know, slimey, eh? So I tell her, "Put ‘em in my dress. Put in my dress." I hold my dress out, I wrap ‘em up all in my clothes and run up. Oh, the water climbing back, you know. I say, "Hurry up, Puanani." The water was coming up, but the kind ripples like. Oh boy, lucky we was far enough already. Lucky the policeman never see. So we went home with the fish. Sarah said, "Where you guys get that?" We tell, "Down the sand." Oh she was mad at us. She know it's dangerous. She said,"You folks might not be lucky." But we was watching the water and picking up the fish. So we had a big party that night. Sarah said boil one squid. We had cooked squid and we had the fish.

And then for a whole week, we fish. We come pick up the fish at the baseball field, cause the water was above our knee. We just go get the wire. So we string all the fish on top the wire and then we tie ‘em up, we get two like that. And then we come home, we give ‘em to the old folks. They tell, "Oh, thank you, thank you. Where you get this?" We no tell where, we say, "Down there. Get plenty more." Had äholehole inside, had menpachi, had po‘opa‘a, had all kinds of stuff inside there.

You see, God caught us all off guard. Even his creatures in the ocean was caught off guard. So that's why I say nobody know when He's coming. You see what he did? He showed us. Not even the fishes know. So we not going know when He come, when you too busy doing something. They say nobody knows when He's coming. Nobody. But all those people that die, they know. They know what's going on in heaven, but they cannot talk. They cannot warn us. The only friends can help us are the grasshoppers, the lady bugs, all the flying creatures. When they fly on you all day long, they trying to tell you something, you know? Sometime it's good news, or bad news.

So we went fishing for a whole week. We take all the best fish. The ones was left behind was hīnālea, and puhi [eel], all the kind we nevah like. So some guys was catching 'em for their cat. They say, "Oh, my cat like this." So they pick 'em up, put 'em in a pan, they take 'em home. They were alive yet, you know. So they put 'em on the grass and they call their cat. "Pussy, pussy." The cat come and eat the fish we never like. And then it started to get stink. The water went down to the ankle [level] and then it was stink. All the rest died, yeah. And the kokuas [government workers] had to go clean up all the dead stuff, put it in the rubbish truck and cut all the grass that wen rot and all that. Then the stuff wen kind of dry up.

Boys and Girls at Kalaupapa

When Jubilee [my husband to be] came out here [1944], he was new life to Kalaupapa. All the boys follow him around because he had new things to show, new things to teach them. You know? If you stay here long time you don't know nothing. The same thing year after year. But when my husband came, oh boy, everything change. They always wanted to do what he did. The boys of Baldwin Home, they all liked what he had to show them. But my husband was advanced in a lotta stuff. He thought they were just like children when he came, they stay with their hand tied. What he knew was a lotta what adults know, cause he was out with people who were getting ahead, and not staying behind like Kalaupapa. So when my husband came the boys was happy. Just like he was a savior. Oh, I tell you, he just changed their life. He had a bicycle, he turned the handle forward, everybody turned their handle that way. You loosen the screw and just turn it forward. And the other part was, he raised the seat the highest it can go so he was sittin just in the front part of the seat. That made him look taller. The boys all liked that idea. He cut his fender short behind, put the red light way up. Everybody cut theirs. And he painted his bike nice, and painted a white mark [line] on the tire. Everybody, all of them on the road, showing off their bicycle.

And he taught the boys new songs, and they would sit together and they have four song. "We are the boys of 299." He was in the army, so he sang that song. And then "Sweet Adeline" and "We're the boys around the corner." That's for Gulick Avenue [in Honolulu], where the corner, the boys all like to sit over there and sing. Cause traffic was not like today. Before, you could sit down by the corner with your leg on the road. Not today.

You see, he was sort of the leader. They admired everything he stood for. He was a tough guy, had a skull and cross-bones on his jacket. Jubilee was a rough, tough bugga. Somebody come up and touch him, pau, he bust 'em. He don't want nobody touch him. They were scared of him. But later on he changed his way around. I admired him very much. I said, "This guy is for me." I saw he was rugged, that's the kind I looking for. I never wanted to go with the boys up here. They were like my brothers. I played with them growing up; I don't wanta sleep with them.

And then us girls, we bought bicycle. Bicycle cheap before. $56. So all the girls bought our bike and we learn how to ride. Then we ask Sarah if we could ride, go out of the compound. She said yeah. So we got up early in the morning, like 2:00. We got on our bike with our flashlight on. All us going down the road. We follow each other, we go down the airport, turn around, come back to town. Once somebody saw us from Baldwin Home. They went home, tell the boys. "You know the wahines, they ride early in the morning. They go on bicycle." Oh! All the boys bought one bike. And pretty soon there was not only us on the road, we saw other headlights coming. You know, it was the Baldwin boys. They wanted to go with us—airport. We never like. Because they good riders, eh? They ride fast. We ride slow. So more early we go. And then we hide. We see their lights coming, so we hide from them in the lane. And they think we went down the airport. We see they all pass us going down towards the beach, we get on our bike, we go back in town. And then by the Mormon Church, somebody said they see the light coming back, so we go behind the shop. That's how we do all morning, hide from them. And they cannot find us. And they get angry. So, when they come visit us, they tell, "Hey, where you guys was?" "Around." "Gee, we look for you, we cannot find you." We say, "We get secret place." "Yeah? Well next time we going be ahead of you guys." "Okay, you go ahead of us." We don't go that morning, we stay home. "Hey, we never see you guys." "Oh, we never go today." "Oh yeah?" Oh boy, we had so much fun with the Baldwin boys. You see, the Catholic boys at Baldwin Home and the Catholic girls at Bishop Home, just like we all close together. So we got along. McVeigh Home and Baldwin Home never got along. They jealous.

Baseball

Baseball, we had the three unit homes—McVeigh Home, Baldwin Home, BayView Home. Cause Bishop Home only girls, they don't play, yeah? And then we had the Outsiders.[10] They challenge each other—the unit home, outsiders; another unit home, the outsiders. Like that. And the girls always root for Baldwin Home, because that's where the Brothers take care the boys and the Nuns take care the girls at Bishop Home. So we always kinda stick together, yeah? And come time the Baldwin Home gotta play Outsiders, or McVeigh Home, then we root for the Baldwin Home boys. Well, most of us had boy friends in Baldwin Home. And we go down there, "Ray, ray, ray for Baldwin Home." And the other guys on the other side, "Ahh, shut up!" You know, they yell at us like that. We get mad, you know, some time just like we like fight. But we let it go. We just down there watching the game, and we get good fun.

And Paul Harada, he was for McVeigh Home I think that time,

[10] The "Outsiders" were those who lived outside the four unit homes.

and he cannot hold the bat [because of his disabled hands]. So they took the innertube, they cut it about three inches, and they left the bat tied on his hands, so when he hit the bat, the bat don't slide. But he hit the ball. Then he was taking off the rubber for run. No can. They say, "Run like that. Run." So finally, he start run. Oh, we just bust out laughing. Everybody in poor condition like that, yeah? We understand. We just get good fun. And then first base when he can take the bat off. And then somebody take 'em back to the home base, the next guy come on.

And you know, we had so many people that time, that baseball field had all cars around the field to the road. Filled with cars. And somebody running home for home run, yeah? So everybody tootin their horn. And the guys that don't go, they say, "Oh, somebody get home run." They can hear the horn. Ohhh, those days are gone forever. All those that were here, all gone.

The Raiders were the best team. It was the one my husband belong in. The best batters were my husband, Nicky and Piko. My husband Jubilee, he wen hit one. Ohhh, over the cattle guard. Way inside the bushes. Oh boy, everybody was steal base. Everybody came home one time. Oh my goodness, everybody wen toot the horn. Yeah, the Raiders were the best players. When they won, all the boys say, "Hey. Get on the car. Follow me." So, we wait till everybody go home. Then long line, Baldwin Home, long line. All us girls with the boys. We going up McVeigh Home first, cause they sore losers. We go up McVeigh Home, they block the road with the rubbish can, all line up. Our boys jump outta the car, pull the can on the side. "Okay, let's go." We go through the McVeigh Home. Toot, toot, toot, toot. Everybody tooting their horn. Oh, these guys they look at us, they so sad because they lose, yeah? And we were the winner, the boys were the winner. And they say, "One more time." We go back inside. Oh, those guys mad with us. Then we go, we yell at them, "Bye, bye." We go to the next home, Bay View. So happy to win, yeah? After that, we all end up down the bar. Sunday they cannot sell beer, but the owner give the beer. He say, "You guys win. Here." He give us the case beer, we go under one tree, suck 'em up.[11] Good fun. Just happen the owner liked the team. That's just how he was. He never cared for the McVeigh Home. They always high makamaka [stuck up]. But he like the Baldwin boys.

And then when the boys win Bay View Home, they go up the road there too. but the bugger they like fight. Cause they older men there. Go up there, go around maybe three, four time. They get mad, they throw the chair from the porch. "Get outta here." Everybody laugh on the car. Ohhh, we had good time before. So much fun. But all of them are dead.

Dating

There were a lotta things we didn't know how to do, yeah? Cause we came here all innocent. But you learn fast over here. You gotta grow up fast, because there's so much things going on. Those days we had nothing but fun. Every end of the month we had a dance in the hall. Anybody they could get to play music, put 'em up there. You know how much they pay? Five dollar each. And our patients, they play music. They had a piano player, they had traps [a drum set]; they had bass, guitar, 'ukulele. And that was enough to make music. We was always happy for the dance; we get to dance with the boys.

Luckily we had Sarah to watch over us. She always said, "I don't want you folks going around. You like go down, you have four guys go one time. But not alone." So that's how we go. Either by threes or fours. And every time when we together, the boys always say "You look like a school of fish." Cause we always together. And she say, "When I say you come home at 4:00, you be sure you home at 4:00." So she had us well covered. Hah, hah, hah! She said, "You folks too

[11] Cathrine was probably around 18 at this time, too young to get beer herself from the bar. Presumably Jubilee or one of the other boys was old enough.

young." But when we got of age, then Sarah said, "Well, sixteen is the right age for dating." But she said, "You know, I don't want you folks to…" "Yes, Sarah. Yeah. Okay. We know." She said, "Behave yourself." Were three girls were old enough to have dates. Had these three boys that took us out. We always watch ourself, if we get too serious, but all of us married them. And then we left home, we went on our own.

I met Jubilee when I was up at the Girl Scout camp. I think I was sixteen. And I didn't think much of him, I used to tell Henry Nalai'elua, "Oh, I hate the looks of that guy." And he said, "Why?" "Look like a criminal." Jubilee and Henry came there to help us. They cut wood for us because we need firewood. And Jubilee's cousin climbed up the cliff. She likes Henry, treat Henry like a big brother. So, Henry was up there already, so she climb up till she reach Henry. She sat down. So Jubilee yell, and he say, "Ka'iu, come down." (Ka'iulani was her Hawaiian name.) "No, I like it up here." But it was steep. If she fall down, she make [die]. So he went climbing up there. He got up there, I could hear him talking to her. "You know, you fall down you make? Come on, let's go down." He brought her down. All the way she nuha [sulky]. He got down with her, he say, "You stay down here. No go up there. Dangerous." Bad nuha. So, he was sitting down and she was making lunch—she and I work together—and she said, "Go give this to Pä'ele [Darkface]." Pä'ele was her cousin, that's Jubilee. Pä'ele means black. Jubilee was dark, yeah? She mad with him, she don't wanta go talk to him. So I say, "Okay." I took it to him, I say, "Here's your lunch." I never feel anything yet for him. Then I look at him. He had a beard, you know? So I said, "Why don't you shave that off? You look like a billy-goat." And he didn't say much about that.

And came the next day, and one of the scout masters saw. She said, "Ah Fong, Ah Fong" cause that's what they call me. I say, "What?" She said, "Oh, I don't know, but something is up." I say, "Why, what happened?" She say, "You better take a look at Jubilee's beard." I look, I say, "Oh, it's gone." She say, "I think he likes you." She kept teasing me. I say, "Naw, I don't think so." But I never really cared, you know.

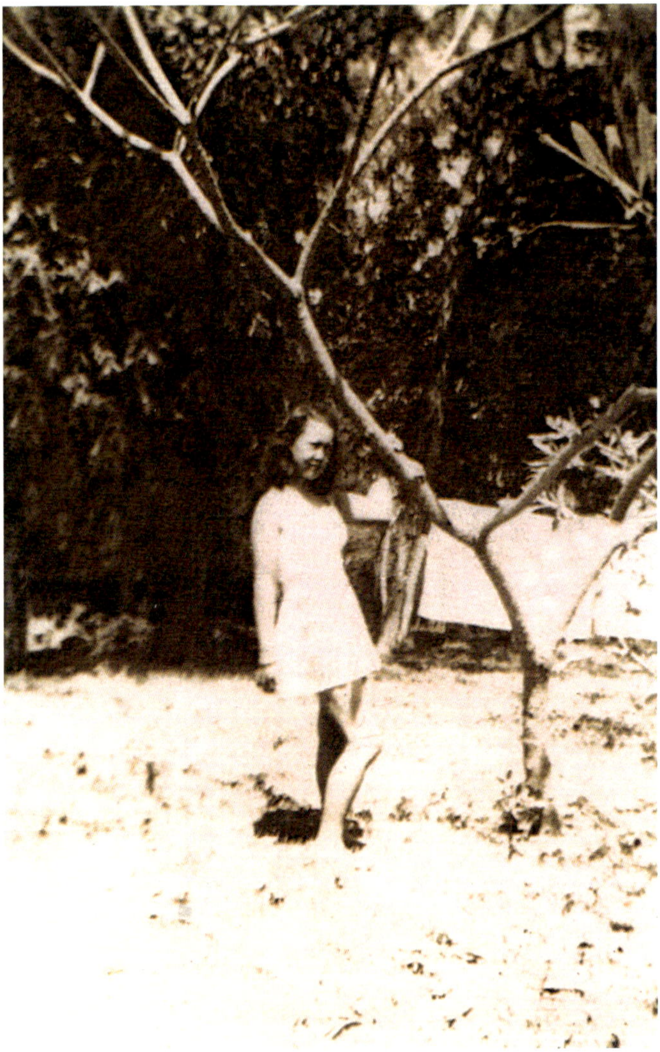

Cathrine at 16, "Posing" (unknown photographer)

That very afternoon he came in my tent. He told his cousin, "Hey, beat it. I like talk to her." "I like listen." He said, "You get outta here before I kick your 'okole [rear end]." She go, "Rahh." So she took off.

So he sat on the other cot, and he was talkin to me. He told me, "I going ask you something. Don't you laugh at me." So he told me he wanted me to be his girlfriend, and he'd be my boyfriend. And I bust out laughing. I thought it was silly. You know, I wasn't in the mood for do that, that feeling was not there yet. He was upset with me. I say, I go home and ask Sarah. Then he said, "You have to tell Sarah?" I tell, "Of course. She takes care of us. We tell her everything." He said, "Everything?" I said, "Well, what are we gonna do?" You know, innocently I talking to him like that. He's two years older than me. I said, "Wait. Let me talk to Sarah." So, he said okay.

I came home, then we had 'ohana.[12] All the girls came back from the camp, cause we's gonna have movies that night. And so I told Sarah after 'ohana, I say, "Sarah, Jubilee wants me to be his girlfriend, and he'll be my boyfriend." She look at me, she said, "Yeah?" I say, "Yeah." Now all the girls all ears, all of them like know. She said, "Well, what do you feel about him?" I said, "Well, I think he's okay." She said, "Well, you're sixteen, you know. Just don't do anything wrong." You know, she's tellin me that.

So I said, "Okay." So that's how we had our first date. When we came back from camp, I tell him, "I can do date with you." He say, "Yeah?" Oh, he was so happy. So we just walk all on the road, walk up and the rain start coming, I say, "Hey, we're going get wet." So we go down the pavilion down at the pier. And we sit under there until the rain pau and we talk sweet nothings. (laughs) And all the girls would be on the porch looking for me. I come home, I told Jubilee, "All the girls are still up." He said, "Yeah, they're looking for rubbish on your hair." I say, "What?" He said, "That's what they do." Even him, when he go home the boys look for rubbish on his hair. You know, they think he's had a rolling session or something. So we go home, he do this, run his hand over his hair, make sure nothing. So I said, "Oh, I don't care. I don't have anything on my hair." Coming home, I say, "Hi," they say

---

[12] See p.14 for the daily service that they called *'ohana.*

"Hi." They looking if my flower all mussed up, my hair all mussed up. And they stand up and they look around me, you know. I say, "What you looking for?" They say, "Nothing." They look all around, they say, "Her hair okay." And they look at Sarah, the girls. Yeah, always tell on each other. Oh, golly. And then the nuns would come out--they see us walking—and say, "Be sure to take a long coat. It's cold tonight." And Jubilee, he say, "Oh well, I'll warm her up." I tell, "Don't say things like that. They'll lock me out."

And then another girlfriend of mine, she had a boyfriend too. But not all the girls had boyfriends. There was about eight more young girls, they always got jealous when we went out on a date. "What'd you folks do? Where you folks go?" They like know everything. We say, "We just walk around. And we not telling you any more." (laughs) They're like our little sisters. Even if we going sneak out, they wanta go too. We say, "No, you cannot go. It's just for us older girls," I say, "No jam us up." We go down the beach, we have a picnic. We had good fun, our innocent days.

I think it was in 1945 we start dating each other. By then I was outta school. Sometimes we would go up to the uncle's house and we cook, and then we had dinner. And he told us, "You folks can stay here." You know? Who wants to stay over there. We wanted to be by ourself. I said, "No, we're gonna take a walk." "But where you folks go?" Hoh, like it was their business. We never asked them where they went. So we just said, "We go down the pier, and sit by the pier." And then we get up, and go walk around the road. We just walk around. We have to go home by 10:00. Maybe we see the other couple walking too, going the other side. We walking with two other couples, because we're old enough to date. It was Puanani and Danny, Annie and Nicky, and me and my husband Jubilee, was going together that time. And some nights at the end of the month we had dances for the settlement. We look forward to times like that. And the boys always tell, "You tell my girlfriend, I going come pick her up." So the boys, they get runners they call 'em, come up Bishop Home. "Hey, you know, Jubilee say they going come pick you up, you know. So you better be ready." "Okay." Then the other kid come for the other girl. They smart, you know. They don't tell us themselves, they have runners. So, we gotta walk. Those days no more car like today. Even the policemen don't have cars, they gotta walk beat.

So, this go on and on and on with the dates, and then come the day when Sarah tell us she's gonna get married. Oh, we was all in shock. "Sarah, you gonna leave us?" We never think about how she feel, we was thinking about how we felt, we gonna lose her. She said, "Yeah. He proposed to me." Then we start to cry. She said, "I'll see you folks around. The older girls can take care of the younger girls." Sarah was in love. She only touch a door, the light would come on, that much current was going through her. Then the day came when she planned to get married. She had a little party on her porch, and only us girls was invited, cause the house was just small, yeah? We had a nice party. Then some of the girls said, "We better go home. Too late already." So we kiss her and we hug her, then we say goodnight. Then we went home, Bishop Home. We went in the house. Feel so empty. We felt like baby kittens that the mother abandon.

After she got married, oh boy, we had a ball. All us older girls got together. "How much you get?" "Oh, I get dollar." "I get 75 cents." "Fifty cents." We put all our money together, we walk down the bar. We call somebody older, we give the money to buy us one bottle wine. "You guys can?" "We're on our own." "Okay." "No tell 'em for us." Baimby they come outside. "Get this one, that's all the money can buy. Port wine." We took the bottle home, and then only the older girls can drink. The young girls sit down, watch us. Oh my goodness, we got so drunk. That wine made us sick. And we said, "Never again."

And then we had a small, short nun, and she always wen check up on us. So we put the dog by the step. She scared of dogs. She come out, "Hello girls. Are you alright?" The dog go, "Rrrr." She say, "Oh no, doggy, no, don't bite me. I don't want you bite me." And we say,

"Get 'em, get 'em." The dog go, "Rrrr." She take off home. After that we leave the dog over there. She don't come in the house, she only check on us, what we doing. We call her Minnie Mouse. She's the shortest Sister I ever see. She know we never cared for her. Says, "Hello girls," and we say, "Oh, Minnie Mouse," and walk away. She always like make good with us. And then somebody say, "Minnie Mouse coming." They all hide everything what they was doing.

I remember the time the girls were buying bicycle. I was maybe sixteen years that time, and my brother asked me if I like one bicycle. You know, lady kind. Those days bicycle only sixty-five dollar. So, I say yeah. So he paid every time to the guy who sold it to us. And then had two more payments left, he came blind. And I just started to go with Jubilee. And he told Jubilee, "I going be blind pretty soon. Can you help my sister pay for that?" And Jubilee paid it up. But I was so embarrassed. I never told my brother do that. Oh, I got upset with him he told me that. I say, "Why did you go ask him?" I say, "I could have paid it." I was growing up and working by then. They gave us job when I was seventeen. We worked in the Bishop Home kitchen and infirmary with the old folks. But he said, "It's alright, it's your boyfriend." I say, "Yeah, but I shame."

And, you know, we got older we gave up the bike stuff. Then we went for cars. Sarah got married already. So we was all on our own. So all the older girls got together and we plan things that didn't include the younger ones. They overhear, say, "I like go, too." And then, "No you guys cannot go. You folks too young." So only the older ones they did, the ones they was 16, 17, 18. Jubilee was the ringleader. He got one car, he told us, "You folks like go picnic?" "Where?" "By the beach." "Okay." I go and tell the girls. He said not until 10:00. 9:00 we was waiting for them. He was upset with me. He said, "I said 10:00. Now the nuns not even sleeping yet." And then he say, "Okay, I take you girls first." He took us down, he dropped us by the beach, then he brought the boys down. And then we had a bonfire, with the hot dogs and all kind stuff for eat. Potato chips, fruits. Then we stayed down there. And had this big mast, from the Ka'ala, the boat,[13] the thing just fell off the boat. And each time it roll in. The high waves brought it right to the sand. So we put kerosene on some parts of it and we lit it for bonfire. And those days the policemen no more car, they gotta walk. And they don't wanta walk way down there so we were safe. Hardly any cars passed by, cause never had cars. When we came home, the nuns wen go check all our rooms, we wasn't in. Called the administrator. The administrator was a Mormon elder. He call all the Mormon girls down to the office, he went for them. Had about five Mormon girls with us, the rest was Protestant. But we never get scolded, we got punish. The nuns wen punish us, said all you folks are not going to the movie for a long, long time. We said okay. So we stayed home, until one day the sisters come and say, "Okay, you folks can go to the movie." Well, by then we was all ready to fly the coop. You know? Those days were not you 18 and you old enough, you gotta be 21. So we had to listen.

Jubilee never end up in jail. Only he did one time over here. Not only him, had five boys and one girl. They took off up the pali trail, and they not supposed to. Cause they were still active case. They all ended up in jail for forty-five days. But they thought that was funny, you know? Because they were all young, and it was exciting. something different. And then when we go to the movie,[14] they all like, "Yoohoo," they clown around. And then the cops used to tell, "Okay, quiet down, quiet down." Anyway, there's lotta them so they talk story, they joke around. And then we can go up to visit them. That time we were just starting to go together. He was about twenty, and I was about eighteen. And they stayed there forty-five days and they came out. It went so fast, just like they stayed only two weeks. But they never went back again, because they start growing up, yeah?

---

[13] The boat Ka'ala had shipwrecked on the reef years before and the mast had floated in to the shore.

[14] The jail was right cross the street from Paschoal Hall, where the movies were shown.

When you start growing up, you don't wanta do something like that again.

When Sarah got married, that left us alone. But we three were old enough and Sarah taught us how to behave ourself and do what is right. So we went on and on and on. And Jubilee told me, "Why don't we get married, so we don't have to go around like this?" I said I have to hear him say one word. He said, "What word?" I said, "When both the boy and girl are in love with each other, they always say something to each other." He say, "Oh. I love you?" I say, "Yeah." He say, "You know very well I love you!" So I say, "Okay, let's not get into an argument." He say "Let's get married." So I say, "Oh, too soon after Sarah." He say, "What's Sarah got to do with this? She's married. Now we talking about us getting married." So, he said, "What about September?" [Sarah had gotten married in June.] I said, "September?" "Yeah, September 15." I said, "Let me think about it." He said, "Well don't wait too long." I go home, I talk to my two girlfriend, I said, "My boyfriend asked me for marry him." She said, "Yeah? and when you gonna get married?" I said, "Well he like get married September." I say, "I don't know yet, I gotta think about it." And the other girls said my boyfriend asked me to get married too, Annie and Puanani. They got married before us. On the sly, you know? They didn't tell us they was gonna get married. And then we see them taking their stuff, going up to this house. And then they saw us. "Oh we married already." I say, "My goodness. You guys kept this a big secret." So she [Puanani] must have told her boyfriend we was gonna get married, so they got married. Then Annie told us she gonna get married before us. I was the last one to get married.

Cathrine's Brothers at Kalaupapa

Then I gotta tell about my three brothers. I had four brothers in here [taken into confinement because of Hansen's Disease]. One did not stay. The oldest, half brother [Solomon], he was [only] suspect.

And one of the other brother, Ah Wah, was supposed to go home with him, but he climb the sour sap tree, he fell down and broke his arm. So they kept him back in Kalihi. That's why he remained here at Kalaupapa for the rest of his life and stayed on with my brother Samson.

Samson was blind, totally blind. When I came in '42, he could see yet. Not that good. My brother, he loved the nuns. He loved to talk to them; he liked to be near them. They make him feel good, you know. My two brothers, they hang around the nuns every time. The nuns like them and give them rosary and stuff. They liked the Catholic church, so they joined. It's okay. They're old enough. They wanted me to join Catholic, but I said, "No, I gonna stay Protestant." I was brought up as a Protestant. Went to a Hawaiian church down Waikane [on Windward O'ahu].

My brother Samson worked at the hospital that burned down. He worked as a janitor. And every time he get through working, he had to walk all the way across the beach, go home to Baldwin Home. He come back all the way, early in the morning, so the nun felt pity for him, Sister Mary Joseph. She told, "Samson, I gonna give you a room in the hospital, and I don't care what anybody says. So you don't have to go home. Sleep here. Work here." So that's where his home was. And I used to go visit him in there and I said,"You lucky you can stay here." He said, "Cooler over here. Much cooler." His eyes got worse after that. And then, he was asked to move out of the hospital, because the nun that was his favorite left the settlement. And when the Mother leave the settlement, changes going be made, yeah? So they told my brother he gotta leave the hospital, he cannot stay in there.

After that he had to go Bay View Home.[15] He was blind already. But he knew everything in his room. He was a ham radio operator. He had lotta cards all on his wall from different ham operator. Each one sent their card number—their station and their name. He can use that

[15] Generally the blind male patients were housed at Bay View Home.

without having to pay the telephone bill. My brother was good, even though he was blind. And I used to bring him up here to my house for eat. Those days we had lup cheong, fried eggs, rice.

Samson love to sing. He was a good worker, but between time he go sing, yeah? My brother always, when he get time, pick up his guitar and he just play. He liked to compose. And he composed song, "Sunset of Kalaupapa." The song belong to all of them that they sang it together. There was Willie, Henry, Samson, Orson, and they had two girls sing, Nancy and Shirley. But because they never like do anything, so my brother had it copyright. Cause my brother had a nurse as a friend, she know how to get in touch with people. She played a big part in my brother having song made. And Frank Owens used to come here, and he and my brother got along. The brother of Harry Owens,[16] so he asked his brother to help my brother with his song. Buddy Fo, he was the singer for Harry Owens, he has a beautiful voice. He sang "Sunset of Kalaupapa" and then he told all the people that came to Coconut Grove—that's where he used to play—he told them to buy a copy of the song for one dollar. So, that's how they had money, and with that money, they bought a piano for the settlement.

But you see, Timothy [a patient who played the piano] and the Japanee foreman, they hated each other. And Timothy took a bunch of keys when he went to Honolulu. He's supposed to leave it back. And then they couldn't open without the key for the piano. They locked it because people go there, play, play, play. And then the foreman got the crowbar. Cause we had outsiders came to play piano, but the key wasn't here. Oh, he was going bdak, bdak, bdak, with the crowbar. He broke the piano cover. Everybody was inside there went, "Oh my goodness." But the foreman he hated Timothy, he wrecked the piano. And that was wrong. It cost a lot of money. I shoulda gone up and hit

---

[16] Harry Owens was a mainland musician who was important in creating a hapahaole style of music in Hawai'i, featuring an acculturated Hawaiian-style melody with an English lyric. In the 1930s he was featured on the Hawaii Calls radio show and later on he often appeared on televsion shows from California.

him. Cause my brother worked hard to get that piano for the settlement.

Chuckie [my youngest brother], he was only one and a half, I think, when my mother died. And my brother Chuckie, his fingers was bad, the last one. We call that crab hand. And we know already he had something, a touch of it. When Chuckie came in, Kalihi Hospital was pau, Kalihi closed up. 1950 everybody went Pearl City to Hale Mohalu. He stayed at Hale. And then, my brother and sister wanted him to come up here, Kalaupapa. See, before, he was staying with my auntie, and they treat him mean. He was just coming out of puberty. And one day he came to see me, he had a big black eye. I looked at him, I said what happened to you? He never like tell, because the cousin were right there. Say, "I fell down." He never like tell that my cousins did it. And then I found out later. Then I came and tell my brother Samson about it, that they don't treat him good. He write to the doctors, he said I want my brother come in here. Those days they okay anything. Today you tell them that, they say, "Oh no, no. He cannot go there, it's off limits." In the early fifties, he came with a bunch of kids, and he asked to remain, while the other younger ones went back to school. So my brother Chuckie stayed here and he helped my brother Samson. He lived at Baldwin Home, but he always come down and see Samson [at the hospital], check on him.

My brother Chuckie stayed until the early 60s. He had to leave because he made the girl friend hapai [pregnant]. He was on temporary release, so he could go if he like. But he was messing around our medical technician, she takes our blood, do the urine tests. He hang out over there every day. And then he asked her for a date. And never take long, he tell us she hapai. I said, "Godfarnit you! Now you gotta take care of her." So then she was showing. They had to get out because the state make them.[17] So he was on his own after that. He got a job

[17] At that time, the state put a patient on "temporary release" if the disease had been rendered inactive by the sulphone drugs, and the patient was allowed to live outside Kalaupapa. They had to move out because the state would not allow a patient to

and they got married and they found themselves a place to stay. And then he had his own family.

marry and live at Kalaupapa at that time with a non-patient spouse. And, of course, a child born to them could not stay at Kalaupapa either.

Chapter 3. Early Married Life (1947 to 1970)

I went with him for two years and then we decided to get married. So I said, "I better talk to Sarah." So Sarah told me, "If you folks love each other, and you wanta get married, I don't see why not." You know, I was eighteen. So we went to the office, the two of us. And we told the administrator we wanted to get married, we needed a house. He said they have an old house up there, they'd fix 'em up, they'd paint 'em. And then people start giving us things for the house. Well, my husband was a very good provider. He bought me ice-box, washer, stove, the furniture for the parlor. Somebody must have gave us their old double bed until we had new one. So we got married and we stayed in that house.

My brother Samson was in love with one of the nurses. She was so good to me. I think two years before I got married [while Jubilee and me were courting], my brother gave her some money one time to buy me shoes and gown for New Year. And she went shopping at Ritz Department Store, Fort Street [in Honolulu]. She said they had a terrific sale. She bought two--one was white, the other one was pink. She say they was so cheap, only fourteen dollar. So I wore the pink one to the New Year's dance. And then when I got married, I wore the white gown. I kept it. And I was smaller than the gown, so I gave it to Y, she can sew. And she made it narrow for me and she cut the sleeve. And then she started to try it on, fit me just right. Well, that's my first marriage, so I took advantage of the white for first marriage. I had about eight crown-flower lei for my head and about sixteen crown-flower lei from my neck down to my knee. You take the outside petal off, just leave the flower head. That's what I got married in, with that white gown.

I never asked my brothers to come. I never asked the girls to come. They know I was getting married, but I say it's a small wedding, nothing big. We were supposed to have a big wedding. Jubilee's uncle was gonna have a big luau. But he interfered with our plans, so the Reverend Alice told him, "Are you getting married?" He said, "No." "Then, let these two children do what they like. They wanta get married now, let them get married now." So he bowed out. We never had no party. His mother and sister came the following week. The uncle was gonna kill two pigs, and make everything, haupia and all that for Jubilee's wedding. But he never like. He tell, "No, no, I don't

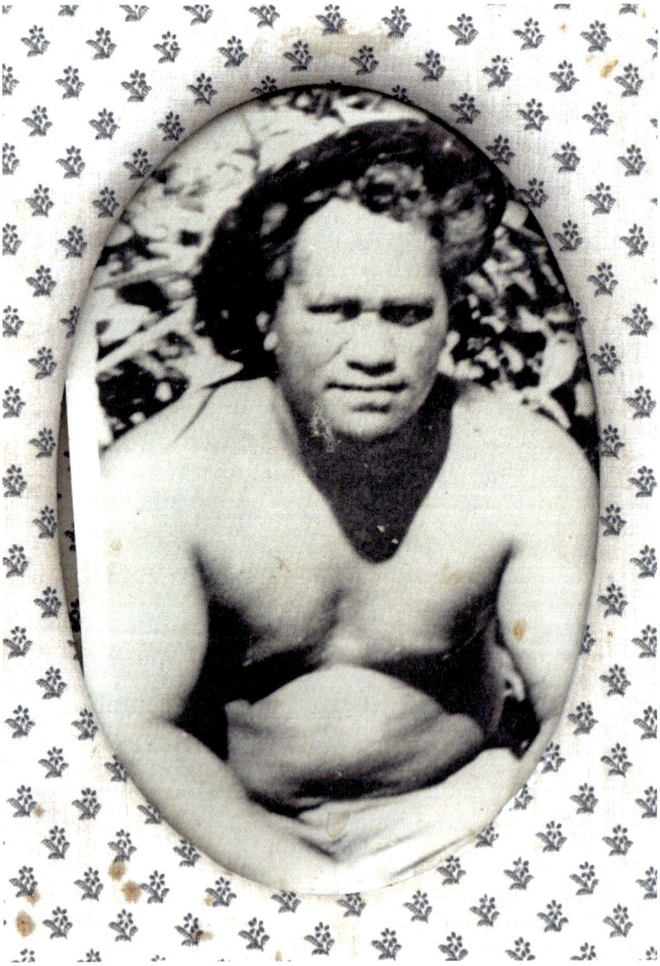

Jubilee at 27, 1956. (unknown photographer)

trust him." Because, you know, when you get married you get things, you get money, yeah? They might think that was theirs because they gave the pig. Just like you gotta pay them back. My husband knew about his uncle them; he said, "No. No party." So what Jubilee and I had for our wedding was can salmon and rice and onion. That's all we ate for our wedding night supper. But just being together was wonderful. You didn't have to hide. You didn't have to run because a car was coming. It was alright.

I burned the rice. You see, Sarah taught us how to cook, but the different girls cook only rice, and the other girls cook the main dish. So we never change over. So I didn't know how much water to put in and it burned. So I started to cry because it burned. So he said, "Oh, let me do it." He threw the rice outside for the birds. He said tomorrow they come for the rice. Then he washed the pot and he made the rice. I was kinda embarrassed my husband had to be the one make the rice, but it turned out real good. We never had table or chair, so we took the coffee table in the kitchen, and we sat on the floor and ate our first meal together. Ohhh, canned salmon. I think everybody had it that was poor like us. Others had chicken dinner, you know. We had canned salmon and rice. That's why I think my marriage lasted almost fifty years. Was shy five months.

Jubilee was a good provider. He was only kolohe [naughty] sometime—I cannot put up with him. Yeah. He was a young man, that's why. But he got over those problems and I forgave him. That's what I think hold our marriage together—I didn't stay mad, I just forgave him. I understood his weakness, and I just let it go. And he came good. I always gave in to my husband when we fought. I let him think he was right, even he was wrong—and most time he wrong. We had a lotta problems, but what marriage don't have problems? But we work at it. We fix it up, we kiss and make up. Well, I just love him. Next year he'll be make ten years. Sometime I eating here, and I look where he used to sit down, yeah? I can imagine where his space, and I talk to him. And sometime I cry. He's not there, but I like to think he's there.

I never drank before. I see him drinking with all the gang, so I start drinking. 1951 I think. I hated beer, but I got used to. I think, if I don't drink with him, I don't get to go places where he go. So I drank. So I went all over. The gang all got together. Annie and Puanani, we all got together, the three of us couples. We went all over party; we go from house to house. We stayed together for a long time. We get through drinking about 3:00 in the morning, we come home sleep. About 4:30 we gotta get up already, get ready to go. Eat, take a shower to go work. And my two animals, I never feed 'em. My dog look at me like this—mad with me. He has that look, "Where's my food?" That's why I figured, I made up my mind, whenever I go out to drink I feed them first.

Daughter Pauline

And then each of us girls had our own life going on. And was not easy. We married too young, yeah? And sometime the husband don't wanta be tied down. He say now I married man, and you gotta give up all that running around and going with the boys. Life's supposed to change. The first time it was kinda hard, he was so used to his single life. He did okay for the first two years, and then after two years I got pregnant. I was married already, so it didn't matter. So my husband was not too happy about having to change his life so soon. Some men get to be hard when they learn this thing, almost like they not ready to be a father. But he had to, because New Year's Eve I was taken to the surgery, and my daughter was born New Year's Day [1949]. But it changed his life. When he saw his daughter, he had a big smile on his face. And he said, "Oh, now I'm a father." I said, "You bet your life you're a father."

When I was carrying my baby, oh my, it was just like a big coconut in my stomach, she was so heavy. And I always craved for sweets. I would give the doctor $10—everything was cheap you know—I said get me a box of chocolates. So I expected a small box. She came back with a huge box of chocolates. I ate 'em all myself. And then another time I was longing for something sweet, I wanted strawberry shortcake. I gave her $10, cause it only cost about $9. She bought me one gigantic shortcake and I ate it all myself. I told Jubilee, I said, "I'm gonna get a daughter." He said, "How you know?" I said, "Girls love sweets." When a boy, when they're pregnant the mother crave for fruits when it's a boy.

I had to go up to Honolulu. My husband took me. I stayed in a building, and next day I told my husband, "Oh, I feel funny." So he told me, "I carry you to the hospital." I said, "Oh, no, no, don't carry me. I'll walk." So, he went up with me. And the nurses told me for go on the bed, lie down. So I stayed in bed until 9:00 in the evening. New Year's Eve. What a place to be New Year's Eve. Instead I'm on the dance floor, I was on the bed in the surgery. I was in bed and I felt my waterbag bust. Oh, I scream, I call the nurse, I said, "I think my baby coming out." You see, all young novice like that, they get scared. And they took me to the surgery and they call the doctor. Doctor talk to the nurses, he say, "Anybody going to any party, cancel all the party, you come stay in here." All the nurses got mad with me. They said, "Just because you we're not going to the luau." Say, "How come doctor wants us all here?" They had to stay in the nurse's quarters all night. I never give birth till New Year's afternoon, 1:30, so they could have gone to their party and come back.

Doctor had a hard time with me. I say, "Doctor, I tired Doctor." I was all dry already. And then he say he gotta call a specialist, he say he cannot do it. So he call Dr. Dixon. Dr. Dixon came, he say, "How long was she in labor?" They said from 9:00 last night to 1:00 this afternoon. He say that's too long, cause the baby could suffocate. So he look at me, he feel, he say, "It is right under your breast. How did it get there?" I said, "I don't know." Then doctor told him that this was my first baby. Then he said, "I have to do this. I'm gonna press down under here so hard, it might feel like my fingers going to go through your skin." He said, "Don't panic. Listen to what I have to say. When I say push, you push with all your might. That's the only way we can get the baby out." And he say, "Okay, are you ready?" I say, "Yeah, doctor." He say, "Okay, when I push, you push." So he went one time he push down on her, and I push one time, that baby went shoot right out. Lucky the nurses was there, with something to catch 'em. She didn't come out slow. But she never cry, so they hold her leg upside down and they tap her 'okole. She never cry, and they was getting scared, you know, maybe she passed away. They listen her heart, she's still alive. So they tap her again, a little harder this time. Then she started go, "Aah-aah-aah." You know? They say, "It's a girl. It's a girl." I always wanted a girl. I always wanted a daughter. And then they clean her up. They suction her mouth, wash her, and put olive oil on top her, wrap her in a blanket. I bought her a pink blanket. "How you know it's a girl?" I said, "I was hoping, so I got pink, everything pink."

And they brought her to me. They said, "Don't kiss her." I cried, you know, I wanted to hold her. They say, "No, you don't touch her." And they went outside—Jubilee was smoking out there—they said, "Look, you have a baby girl." And they said, "Don't touch her. We going take her to St. Francis Hospital." They took 'em away from us right away, see? You cannot touch. The baby stay inside the hospital for one week, and then after the week, whoever going take her come pick her up. And if you try to take 'em to see us, we cannot.

He look at her and he smiled. They said, "Go inside there with your wife." Then he came inside, until they got me ready to take me back to my room. Then he sat down, and every time we giggle, like two young kids don't know what to do. Then he held me, and then he thanked me. He said, "I know you suffered." I say, "Oh yeah, I had hard time. She just wouldn't come out."

So I had given my baby to his uncle because the father and mother never respond. I wrote a letter to the mother that I was gonna have a baby, I had my things for her. We didn't wanta put her in a home, so I figured she could help us. My mother-in-law was sickly. She said, "I cannot, I'm sick." So, we decided to give 'em to his uncle, he wanted one child. I tell them I'm havin a baby and I would like them to take care of it. She [Jubilee's mother] never tell her husband, and when he found out, he was so upset. He said, "That's our first grandchild. I'm going Honolulu." The night before we was gonna make the papers, my husband's father came down, he said, "You know something? Nobody told me I was gonna be one grandfather." He said, "I want my girl, my first grandchild." Then I said, "Daddy, I wrote to Mama and told her, and she said she cannot." "Well the mother never told me anything. I just found out today." So I thought him and his brother was going fight, you know. I never like him take her, but it's so hard, yeah? Oh, I look at him with the uncle, with his brother. He was crying. The uncle say, "Why she never tell you?" "I don't know, my wife like that." He say "Brother, that's not my fault. She never tell me anything. If I knew, if the letter was read to me, I would tell her yeah, tell her I take care." I said, "Please don't fight. It's no good for the baby." They say no good if you fight over a baby like that, because sometime the baby grow up sick, yeah? And then, reluctantly, his uncle gave in and he gave him his grandkid. He said, "Okay, brother, but it broke my heart." He say, "I was all ready to bring her up and make a Christian life for her." But he said, "That's alright, I give her up." He went home. He was crying. He was real disappointed, because they cannot have children. And even the wife was crying too.

And then my father-in-law stayed, with the wife. I say, "You know, I never like this happen. I asked, but Mama never respond." He's mad with his wife. He tell, "Your fault, Mama. You supposed to tell me." Well, I thought she was gonna read the letter to her husband, but she never, she hid it. And then when the baby was born, she was there, my mother-in-law, the one say she's so busy, she's sick. With a big smile on her face. I said, God fun it, through her came all this trouble. And now she looks happy. Then when the baby was growing up, they loved that baby so much, I thought we no going see the baby again. You know, just like they was going take 'em for them. But because the name was the same, I never care. Even if they adopt it, the baby is still a Puahala. You know? But they say no need adopt, because she's with them and they family.

I saw her when she was a little baby. First visit, that was 1949, my husband and I went to Maui. She was, I think, about two or three months; then they allowed us to go on a plane, to go visit her. But we had to stay at the abandoned airport, Kahului, and they had to have a Board of Health nurse there to watch us so we don't touch the baby. She just sit on the car and look at us. We wanted her to disappear so we can have more privacy, yeah? She watch us the whole time. His father and mother were there cause they took care of her. The father was holding the baby, my husband's father. He was so happy, because that was his first grandchild. And there was no place to sit down—no bench, no chair. We stood up the whole hour talking to each other. Then the Board of Health nurse came to tell us that we had to leave, cause it's one hour. Then my in-laws gave me pictures of her—my baby, our baby. And when we got on the plane ready to fly, then I start crying then, after looking at her picture. Oh, I just cried all the way to Kalaupapa. And my husband knew how I felt. He put his arms around me and he held me. Men don't cry; they feel sad. Cause they not like women. You know, we cry for everything. Yeah, I cried all the way to Kalaupapa, cause I felt so bad, have to leave my baby back. People don't know what we go through being separated from our children, our babies. They don't think we had a sad life, but we do.

I get to see her as she grew up, when she went to Honolulu at my husband's uncle's house and we stayed together. She was about six years old that time. A few other times we went back to Maui too, as she grew up. In '59 I was released—temporary release. They call it parole. That's when I stayed with her in Maui.

And then, when she was twelve or thirteen, she went to Kam School [in Honolulu]. I went to Honolulu, and she came up [to see me] on the weekends. Every Saturday you can go get them at Kam School. And she stayed with me at the hotel. I could go [out from Kalaupapa]. My husband couldn't go; he wasn't released yet. So I went out with his uncle and auntie to go pick her up. Or else I would go up with a taxi. And I paid the taxi driver extra money to go in and ask for her. I told my daughter to be waiting around the gate. And he would go up and ask, "Are you Pauline Puahala?" "Yeah." "Well, I have somebody waiting for you in the taxi." And she came back down, there I was in the car waiting. So he would drop us off at the Blaisdell Hotel. It was on Fort Street. We never go any farther than Blaisdell Hotel, because we don't know if they would accept us anywhere else, yeah?

Then I introduce her to her cousins. She had a boy cousin, and he asked me if he could take her to the car races. I say, "Is it dangerous?" He said, "Not really." And my daughter went with him that night. And you know the young, they enjoy anything fast. She told me she had a nice time. But when he brought her home to the hotel, I was fast asleep, cause they came home a little after eleven. I trusted, because she was with her own cousin. And they went to the desk, they wouldn't let her come up. They thought she was lying. They call my room, I never hear the phone ring, I was fast asleep. So, she went home to my sister's house with her cousin. And my sister called, still I didn't answer. So she slept over there with my sister them. And next day, she brought her back to the hotel. And she told the desk that my sister is upstairs, so call. Then I answered the phone. They say, "We tried to get hold of you last night, you didn't answer". "Ah," I told her, "I had couple a beers with some friends. I pass out. So I didn't hear the phone ring." Some of my friends came over, yeah? To visit with me. I think I better not do that anymore.

But I go get her when I can go out and take her out with me. I take her go shopping. She used to get so much things. Specially on the Valentine's Day. My daughter get the red carnation lei, she get a big box of candies—chocolate—and she get a box of long-stemmed roses. Well, I did it for my only daughter. I loved her. I wanted her to be happy, so I did all that.

And then she graduate. Oh, my brother couldn't tell that's my daughter. They look all over for her, you know? So many girls, yeah? She had--at that time the style of the hair was, she make one curl on the forehead. Do you remember that? She had her hair done that way so they couldn't tell it was her. She looked different. And then one of my nieces kept following all the girls, and then she said she think that's her, she call, "Ka'iulani." (They call her by her Hawaiian name.) Then my daughter turn around. And then they go up there, pile her up with all these lei, right up to her eyes. And then, you know? One of my daughter's teacher when she graduate, they look at me, they say she don't look like you. I say, "Of course. I have the sick now." But my daughter Ka'iulani tell, "Ma, I think if you wasn't sick, I would look just like you." And that's true, she and I have the same features.

She graduated in '67, got married '68, got one baby '69. So, we became grandparents. I had only one, a daughter. And she has only one. So that's the only problem, our granddaughter. She supposed to make the children for us. She said, "Nooo." So look, our family cannot grow.

Those days was twenty-one [when children could visit]. When she was sixteen, cannot come. So, we feel we're the losers. There were so many things that happened that made life miserable for us. Today, sixteen they can come. They lucky. We had to wait too long.[18] A lot of them died; they never even had their children here to enjoy.

The first time my daughter came here, she came here with her husband. And we had a party at the beach, Ocean View. We invited all our friends to come and have supper with us. And my son-in-law, he was tryin to keep up with us, cause we are heavy drinkers those days. He couldn't. He got sick the next day, and we had to nurse him back.

[18] Children have always been restricted from visiting Kalaupapa, because they are more susceptible to Hansen's Disease than adults are. Pauline was never able to visit Catherine as a teenager, because in those days you had to be twenty-one before you could visit. Later on the age for visitation was lowered to sixteen.

And he says, "I don't think I can do this anymore." He says, "You guys drink like fishes." It's true. Patients can drink! My husband used to buy four or five cases of Primo. That was the beer those days. Everybody loved Primo. It was island-made, that's why. Too bad they had to give that up, yeah?

Life in the 1950s and 1960s

A lotta things went on in Kalaupapa, lotta nice things. Well, I thought this was a land of milk and honey. We had fishing during the day and then at night we had a big dance in the hall. Every month we had dance, and everybody looked forward to the dance. We had our local people playing. I think they paid only $5 to each player. $5 was hard to come by before, you know, never had that much money before like today. And sometime we had people from Topside19 come down, entertain. The Topside people get little bit more [money]. Dances were once a month, the last Saturday. We get dance for the whole settlement go—doctors and nurses, kokuas, patients. We had lotta patients .We had plenty of them—two hundred, almost three hundred. Plenty on the floor.

Jubilee loved fish with net, especially for kala [unicorn fish]. Everybody in Kalaupapa loved kala They make soup, they make dry, they fry it, they pülehu [charcoal broil]. They can do any kind thing with kala. I think kala was the number one fish. It's so ‘ono [delicious]. You can even sashimi that. With shoyu and mustard. Hoh! And my husband, he was big and strong. And he used to be the one that carry the net. And he walk out and he start setting it. But you have to go until six feet deep, and you start setting it. And he was only 5-8, you know? And he went out with pants—not shorts—because the kala can cut your legs up, and Lucy's husband was the one that tell

[19] From Kalaupapa, you must climb the *pali* to get to the main part of Moloka‘i. For that reason the Kalaupapa people call the rest of Moloka‘i by the name Topside.

him where to go, and come all around [making the net into a half-circle]. So he drop the net, drop the net, till he come inside. And then everybody jump in the water and start splashing. And the men on the sides start pulling in the nets. Oh, you see the fish all going like that in the water. Pull 'em up to the road. Then they hemo [take out] the fish from the net and they get all of this fish. People you never see around was all around then, because they see the fish. But he used to share with those who came down to help pull the net, you know, and take the fish out of the net. All the family had so much fish. I said, "You know how you guys got plenty? Because you guys share." When you start sharing you get more. And they just tell the people, "Help yourself, help yourself." Everybody so happy, they going home and cook their fish.

Kala, those days we just kept the fire going, you know? Guts and all on top the charcoal. And then we turn 'em over. And guys drinkin on the table already, just take 'em and give 'em. Here's your püpü. Oh, they tear the skin and start poking for the meat, it's fresh. They get mustard and shoyu on the side, eat the meat. Ohhh.

In the fifties, early fifties, they started fishing for kala. The kala was always there, but the patients that was here was not able to do it. They had sores on their legs and hands, they couldn't go in the water like the boys of our era, yeah? Their fingers good, their hands was good condition, they could do it. The people here were old already, cause before they had no young people sent here.[20] So the younger set came in, they could go fishing. They could make wana [sea urchin]. And when they had the akule run, ohhh, they have another one [group fishing with the lay net].

We are so lucky here in Kalaupapa, there is so much fish. Before only the patients could go fishing; the ocean was off limits to the

[20] Generally patients were kept at Kalihi Hospital while they were young and not yet disfigured, then sent to Kalaupapa later. Cathrine and her cohort were sent to Kalaupapa at a young age after the Pearl Harbor attack because Kalihi Hospital lies close to Pearl Harbor and was considered vulnerable to enemy attack.

kokuas. They could only work and stay in their own area. They were not allowed to go fishing or roaming around. They could not own a car. Only the doctors had car. And the delivery car to take the food all over. But kokuas were not allowed.

Moi liʻi [baby threadfin fish] happens in November. Oh, that was a fun thing to do. They are about 6 or 10 inches long, and then they get to be big, you know. So Lucy, her husband John, my husband and me go. John always depend on my husband, because my husband had good feet, good hand, good eye. Cause John never had fingers, his fingers are all sunk in lower than mine. And his feet no good for go in the water, he had bad feet. But he was a good fisherman. So he say, "Oh, moi liʻi running." Oh, get in the car, get all that boxes and everything, and going down the Black Sand. That's where they are [the moi li'i], down the Black Sand. They close to the shore. Because the big fish chase them, and they scared, they stay there close to shore. So John see ʻem already, he tell me and Lucy, "Hey, you two guys go down there and we going set the net over here, Jubilee and me. When I tell splash, you guys splash, yeah?" Hoh, they go all in the net, and then they drag ʻem up to the sand. And that's not all of it, now. You fill a bucket up, set again. Then we see this guy coming. And he like fish; he going ask us for fish. So we dig a big hole and we bury the bucket full of fish [to hide it]. And then, you know, we never find it again. God wen punish us. You see, we should have kept a marker on—somebody's shirt or shoes on top. We didn't put a marker. After the guy left they had to dig, dig, dig. All the sand full of holes, we couldn't find it. What we should have done was let the dogs sniff it out, they can smell better. We were always afraid of that Chinese man. He was a elder to the Mormon church. And you know, he never satisfied, he want more. Yeah, that got us so angry so we bury the fish. We never did that again, ever. We say next time he come, give ʻem. We learn one lesson, never to do that again.

That fish was easy, cause when you start moving them out the scales come off. You don't have to scale it, the scales fall off. So what we did was, Lucy and I took it home, and roll 'em in flour, and she fried it. She fried the whole thing, guts and all. And you know, after couple beers, taste good. Crispy. You just stick 'em in your mouth and crunch, right through the scale.

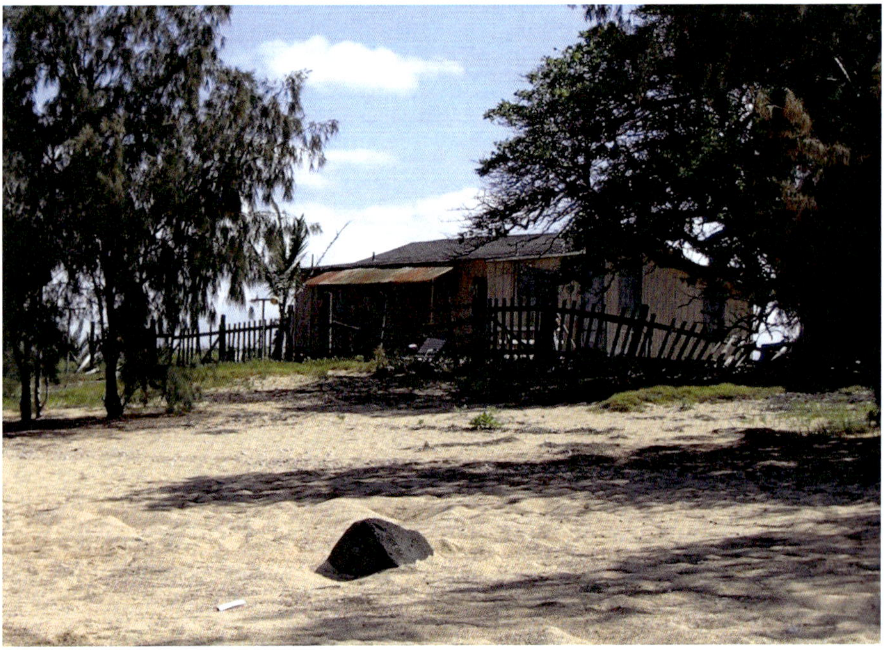
Beach house at Kalaupapa, 2006. (photo by C. Langlas)

We used to stay down the beach house. Cause my friend loan us the beach house, so we took care of the place. It's so good to go stay down the beach. Early in the morning you can hear the water coming in, going out. Nighttime you can hear the water rising, coming inside. There's an old stone wall out by the beach houses, goes out into the ocean from shore. We used it for catching 'upäpalu [a small lavender fish with an orange stripe]. It's just like a stone wall, but it's not that high. We go to fish when the tide is low. Then you could go way out. That wall been there ever since we came. When the tide is so low, you can stay out there maybe half hour, then you gotta keep lookin at the tide, yeah? coming up. Covering the rocks in the front already. So you try catch as much as you can, and then you better start coming home quick. Cause you don't know what inside the stone wall get. I always go with my long boots.

I caught 67 'upāpalu one time. I gave the fish to the old people, cause the flesh is soft. They no get teeth, but they could gum it. They tell me put salt and chili on the fish, then let 'em miko [absorb the salt]. You know, they say "'Ono. Thank you." They love their fish with salt. Easy for them to eat. They eat everything, head and all, cause the bone is soft. I love to go catch that. It's so easy. You wrap the cord around your finger. You use squid bait, eh? let it go down in the hole. And you watch, you see the fish come up. And then some time the puhi [eels] come. They come up and they open their mouth. You say, "Wahhhhhhhhh." That is so ugly, eh? Oh, I scream, I move. I don't stay over there.

I used to have a cat, I put 'em on a rubber raft, an air mattress. And I pull 'em out with me and go out. Not too deep, you know. I pull 'em around. The cat would stay on it. Oh that cat is so unbelievable. It would stay in our car by the windshield sleeping, the car going all over the place. But we killed it by mistake. We used to take 'em down the beach house, but we left him home, we didn't bring with us down the beach. And he heard our car coming, he ran to the car. I told my husband move the car up, and he let the car roll back. The cat was under the tire. Oooh. He ran the cat over. Broke my heart.

Anita. She's Korean. She was a beautiful girl. When I went in to Kalihi, I was about nine. I saw her. And me, I was attracted. I like look, I like follow. She tell me, "What you following me around for?" I tell, "You look like the kind girl in the circus." You know, the side-shows. My father used to take me circus every time. Side-show, they get girls all make up, you know, they beautiful. And they had all this nice clothes. And Anita used to put on Maybelline lipstick, eyelashes, and she used to be so pretty. She never like me follow her around, until

I tell her why I follow her. I tell, "You so pretty." You never can tell she's sick. She just had a little mark on her arm. The rest of her body was just fine. And I think she stayed two years [at Kalihi], then they were sent to Kalaupapa. When we came, few years after that, I couldn't believe that was Anita. I look at Anita, I said, "Anita?" She said, "Yeah." "That's you?" She said, "Yeah." She was all changed, her face, from the beautiful girl I saw. Her face different.

I used to go her house every time. She and I were drinking partner. She call me up. "How 'bout a cold one? Come on over." I go out back. She and I visit, drink, drink, drink. Then she tell me, "Oh, you sleepy?" I tell, "Not me." "You can drink one more, yeah?" I tell, "You better believe it." I feel like I only had two, but I had six. But one thing with her, she make pupu before you drink. If you think you feeling like your head going around, start eating, and that will hold you on longer.

I used to have girl friends. We drank to 4:00 in the morning. Oh, we had good fun. I tell, "Hey, my house tonight." "Okay." "What I going bring?" "Bring salad." We all come together with all the kaukau [food]. I feed my husband first. I tell, "Go in the room, look TV." Then I can be with my girlfriends. Oh, we get good fun. They all make. My best friends—drinking friends—was Shirley and Juggie. Shirley died from heart trouble. She drank too much. She smoked too much. I tell her "Stop smoking." "No, I like smoke."

Smoking, I only fool around. My husband tell me, "Get the hell outta here." I used to go outside on the porch. But I stopped. I had to go hospital for five months. I had bad sickness, and the doctor told me I could get TB. He told me, "Lucky you came in." I could have died. So I stayed in the hospital, and he tell me, "You smoke?" I tell him, "Just for fun. Just fool around." He said, "Don't smoke. It can kill you." So I stopped smoking. I never did smoke again. But I still drank.

I always wanted to be a psychiatrist. I don't know why. I guess because I lived with the same people for years, I know their in and out, everything. But if was somebody else, I think I would have a hard time, yeah? And sometime, I feel like there's some kinda magical powers come to me for some reason, just give me a little knowledge of what's happening. And a lotta time it's just guess work, you just lucky. One time my husband told me he's going out to the beach house. And two wives came to see me, they wondered where their husbands were. I said, "Who were they with?" Then I figured out they had all gone down to a beach house with three girls. They were all drinking at the bar and then they went out there. So we went down there and found our husbands and we had a big ruckus. We got our husbands and came back. When we came back they told me, "How you knew?" I just knew where they would go that late at night.

Deaths

My girl friend died 1953. That's the year my brother Ah Wah died. And my father died same year. We went down to Honolulu for Jubilee to get medical treatment and we was down there. So when my father died, I call on my youngest brother Chuckie. He's like nineteen. I told him, "You go home to Kalaupapa with brother Ah Wah." (That's the one died.) And you go home with brother Samson. (He was staying at Hale Mohalu then for treatment, and he was ready to go home.) I told Chuckie, "You take brother Samson home and Ah Wah. We cannot go home, cause Papa going die next." He say, "Okay, I take them home." So he escorted my blind brother and the dead brother. I say, "You take care everything yeah? You can. Samson can help you." I talk to my brother, he say, "Yeah I help. No worry." I say, "Papa going die. He's tired. So I going stay down, with my husband." So my father died one week to the day that my brother died. So me and my husband stayed for the funeral. After that, then we went home. Everybody was talking, "How come you folks never come bring home Ah Wah?" People here are just really nosey. I say, "Look, my father was dying. I had to make the choice." I said, "It's not good we come home, then we gotta go back again. It's too much for Jubilee to travel that much. He's just getting better." I said, "We had to stay till all pau." Then when they buried my father, then we came home.

Chapter 4. Later Married Life (1970-1996)

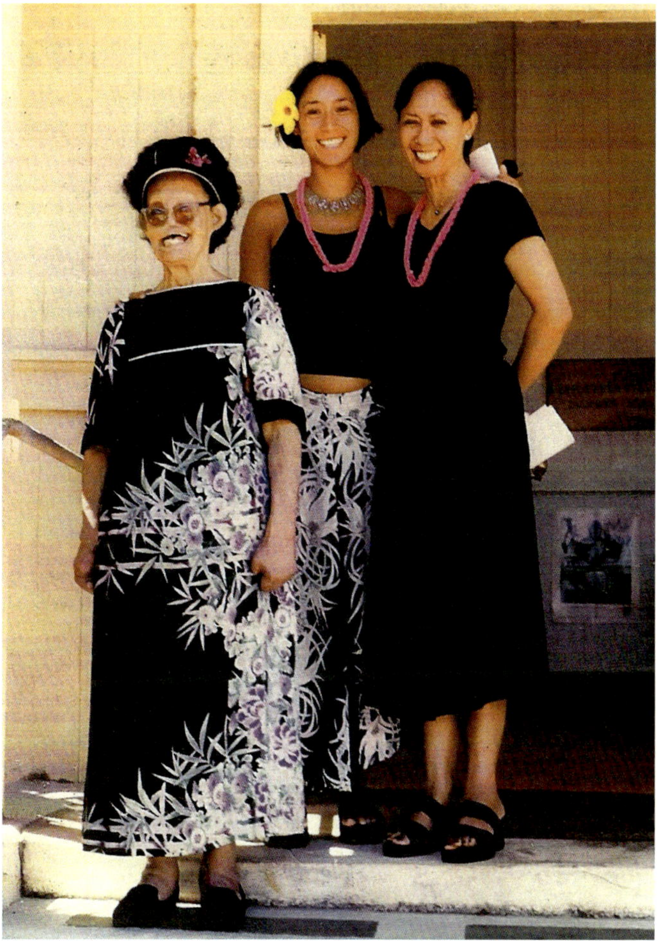

Cathrine, with daughter Pauline and granddaughter Haunani, c. 1985
(photo by Ka'ohulani McGuire)

Granddaughter

When she [Cathrine's granddaughter] made sixteen, that was her first trip over [c. 1985]. My daughter and her came. It's the first time she saw me and my husband. She just stare at us. Because they don't see people like us outside. And next time she came back, she got used to us. She don't stare at us after that; she got her fill of looking at us. So, that goes for everybody. When they get used to they just don't bother staring. Yeah?

When she first came up by herself, she came with shorts—you know when you cut the shorts at the bottom, all jagged. She had a hat on, she had a short blouse you tie in the front. Had her little bag. Looked like a kid going fishing. I say, "Oh my, you got some clothes?" She say, "Yes, I have." I say, "Well, this is Kalaupapa. You can dress like that. It's okay." But young kids dress like that outside, like they going to the beach. Then she stayed with us for a whole week. Then she went back out. I was happy to have her here.

And now she's a lady. She not married. Other people have eyes for her. And I told her who and who was lookin at her. And she say, "Grandma, I'm not interested." I say, "Well, someday you have to find somebody. And you find somebody that can take care of you. Don't go find somebody that don't wanta work. How you gonna live?"

Getting Paroled

When the new medicine came out, was '46 I think, they was giving out the new medicine. Oh, there were a lot of drugs. We had promacetin, diasone, promizole. And the DDS and promin. Promin was one of the strong ones.[21]

---

[21] Promin was the first of the new drugs used to control Hansen's Disease, introduced at the National Hansen's Disease Center in Carville, Arkansas in 1941. Soon after, diasone (or DDS), promacetin and diacetyl DDS were introduced in the

I went promin. The nurse gave it to us in our veins. You know, it's best if she go slow, but sometime they shove it in so fast you wanta vomit. My eyes come all blur and I get dizzy. So I told the doctor I don't wanta take it anymore. He ask me why, I told 'em. One guy got it so fast, he walk outside the porch, make! He collapse and died. Because he got it too fast for his system to grab hold of. He died. Oh, when I saw that, I'm not gonna take no more. So they have to try something else. It didn't work for me. Some, it did work for them. But those that took the promin [and] they had large nodules, all on their knuckles, all on their neck, it melted that away. It disappear. All flat. And we all said, look how the medicine help him. He was lucky, he got well with that medicine. For some, no good.

The promizole was a pill—I think it was white. Even the DDS was white. Diasone was orange, but the shape was flat. Actually, all those pills came out almost about the same time. Yeah? The doctor just try this on that person, that on the other person, and see how it works. I think they only tried me DDS. I don't know why. Others were going promizole, diasone, they was going for different one. Me, I couldn't, I had to go the one they said. 1959 they say I could go. They call that temporary release. So I went to Maui, and I visited my daughter. I stayed with her for about a month, and then I came home.

My husband tried promin, and he good for a while, but he didn't stay on it. He didn't like it. They gave us the chance to refuse, or try something else. He did try something else. I think they call it diasone. He was taking that and it did help him. He looked like he was ready to go out. But he like it here so much that he didn't wanta go out. He wanted to spend the rest of his life here. And I'm glad he did, because my husband, he was somebody that don't wanta be told. And people like that get in trouble, yeah? He was always a wild person, gonna do what he want. If you tell 'em you cannot do that, that's what he wanta

early 1940s (Robert Hastings and Diltor Opromolla, *Leprosy*, 2nd edition, 1994, pp. 17-18). All of these are derviatives of dapsone, which was established as the drug of choice by 1950.

do. As long you stop him, he wanta do that. And I know where he would end up, in jail. So I'm glad he stayed back, because he lived a little longer, and he never end up in jail.

And 1968, me and my husband got sick again. I came sick cause I never take my medicine. My husband never thought it was necessary. My husband and I could hardly talk. We were whispering. Raspy voice we had, "Wha,wha, wha, wha." So I said, "Oh boy, I got it back again. I know. It always goes for the throat, this disease." And I told my husband, "We gotta go Hale Mohalu and try ask for the B6." It was a new medicine.[22] It was God-sent. Only thing, that medicine make you so dark you look like you get the plague. So we ask the doctor down there, we like be on the list, we like to try the new medicine. He say, "Well, you folks have to go through lotta tests." They give us a gallon, you gotta fill that whole gallon with shishi. After you fill 'em up, you put in icebox. They had one icebox only for that. And when the gallon was full, they do lotta tests on that urine. I don't know, just red tape I think. And then we had to do other things. And we took the medicine. They gave us three every day. They could have killed us. They said two was enough, three was too much. Ohhh, golly, we broke out in this… Look like we had this mange. And it all was so itchy. So when we see the doctor, I say, "Doctor, look at me." They said, "That's what we were waiting for. We were waiting for what's inside to come out. Now it's coming out." So they treat us, treat us, and then all this stuff start to disappear. All this dried up, on the surface, you know? They gave us cream, cause we were really uncomfortable. Finally it went away, and our skin started to look good. But, oh, we went dark, dark, dark. I look in the mirror, oh my goodness. Almost look like one colored. That's how much they gave us. But, you know, we took that until 1972. And then 1972, Doctor was taking tests on our skin, check our blood, and make snips and all that. They said, "You don't have any

[22] By 1964, resistance to dapsone was developing (ibid, p. 19). Consequently, B6 or clofazimine, was introduced to control Hansen's disease.

live bugs. They all dead. Nothing is moving, it's dead." Cause they cut some meat out, and they rub on the glass, then they look through the scope, yeah? And they said, "You can go out. We let you go as t.r., temporary release."

But Jubilee couldn't go out, he's still active. But I can go out, so I tell him, "Take your medicine. Listen to them what they tell you." So, he kept taking it. They told him, "You can be a t.r." Oh boy, he was so happy. So, Jubilee became a t.r., and then because I been going out all the time, I kinda knew the place a little bit. So I tell him, "Let's go Blaisdell Hotel." It was a cheap dive. And I told him, "You want so I write?" I make the paper for how many days we going stay, cause I no shame already. The lady was so nice. She seen I had the disease. And she know I write and my husband stay on the side, so lōlō [slow-thinking] like. I say, "You gotta watch me, cause some day you gotta write." So they give us our key. I pay the how much. Then we go on the elevator, we go upstairs. Then they take us to our room. I say, "This is our room." He say, "Oh, not bad." That kind no screen, only window and shade. Wasn't a really nice hotel, but it was where we wanted to be, right close to town. Right across the Catholic church, at Fort Street, Honolulu. You know, all Kress Store and all that on the opposite side, all line up. So, he and I go out. We can go restaurant, and feeling kinda used to. Then when I went Hale Mohalu by myself, Winifred was going to Pagoda Hotel. She tell me, "You like go Pagoda one night with me?" Cause she scared those days, scared stay by herself. I say, "Oh, how much I gotta pay?" She says, "Oh, I paid for it already." She tell me I don't have to pay much. So I say okay. She and I came up, and we stayed at the Pagoda. I say, "Oh, this is nice. Nice look, and nice scenery." You know, that's where I took my husband next. I say, "We go different place," I said, "but you gotta write." He gotta write, cause his hands were better than mine. So, we go by the counter, and they tell him, "How many days?" and he write and sign his name. Then they give us the key. Then they take us to our room. And from that time on he got used to, no shame. Then we go out every

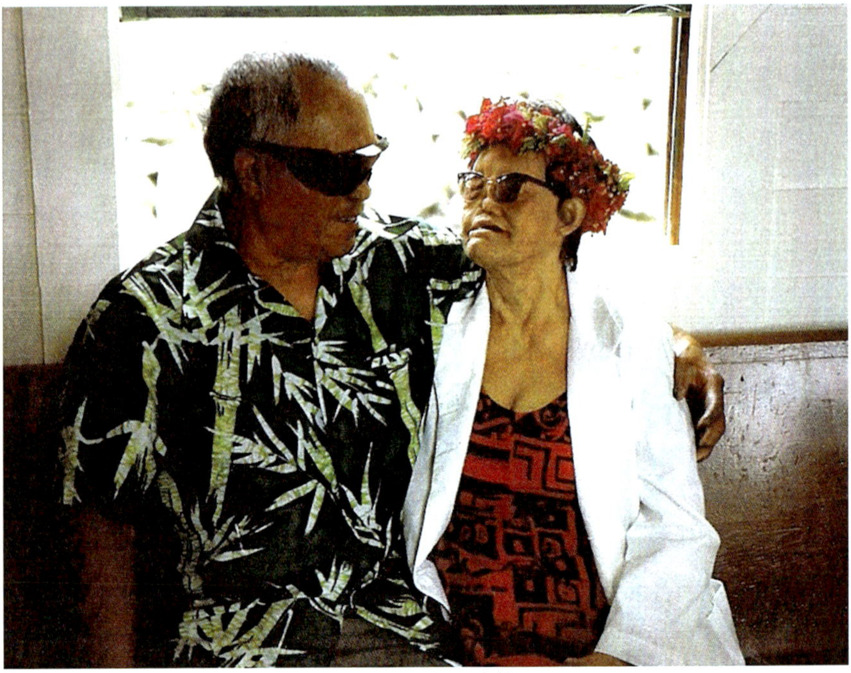

Cathrine and Jubilee.
(photo by Ellen Storm)

time. We go restaurant, we go shopping. We free.

Then we learn about Las Vegas. See M [another patient] told me, "You like go Las Vegas?" "For real?" She say "Yeah. You can go with us." Only she say don't tell my husband. But I did tell him. He tell me, "I like go too." So I went back, go tell 'em, "Jubilee like go too." Oh, their face drop. Because they never like any more go, eh? I say, "If he no can go, I no like go." Cause I no like see him sad, yeah? So they said, "Okay. Okay, we go." Ohhh, that time we went. Next time we catch a plane, we going. We never stopped going. Me and my husband go every time Las Vegas. We work, and then we save our money. We was lock up so many years—like prisoners. Now we get a chance for enjoy.

I still take DDS. Every day I gotta take. The doctors outside they work with us, they want us to be under something. Because they handling us, and outside people meet us, so they want us be under something.

Physical Losses

1976 I went to Carville.[23] I wanted to try build up my nose.[24] I had a plastic surgeon [Dr, Stott] to do the work, that's what he does, but the doctor in the hospital, Dr. Hanna, wanted to do the work. They argue back and forth. And then Doctor Hanna was getting mad, you know, almost he fire the plastic surgeon. So that plastic surgeon kept quiet. He didn't want to be kicked out. Doctor Hanna did it. He didn't know what the hell he was doing. He was going inside, pulling out bone, going back, pulling out bone. The plastic surgeon told him, "Enough, don't take any more bone, she won't be having no bridge." Oh, and he took one too many. So my eye glass every time fall down. Oh, Doctor Stott was so mad. Doctor said, "You cannot hold your glasses up now. It's gonna fall." I said, "Doctor Hanna is like that. Stubborn." So he did what he could, and then, they were dressing my nose, looked big. When it got healed, I took the dressing off. Everyday you could see 'em going down, going down. When I came home, I thought my husband going be happy to see me. You know, with that big nose? He look at me just like, what happen? I say the doctor stubborn. He wanted to do the job and he bungled it. The whole thing. So I never wanted to go back again. They tell me, "You go home, and when you wanta come back, you just let us know." "Yeah, okay." I get home, no more. I said, "I ain't going back."

I had an accident with this right eye. I slept on the floor one night, and then when I stood up, I stood up right by the corner of a wrought-iron table. And it just sliced my eye open. And the fluid was coming out. So I just sat in shock on the chair. I couldn't move, I was so

---

[23] The National Hansen's Disease Center is located in Carville, Louisiana. Many of the Kalaupapa patients went there for specialized medical treatment.

[24] As often happens with Hansen's Disease patients, the bone in Cathrine's nose had shortened, just as it does in the fingers.

scared. And then next day, I went to the hospital so they look at my eye. I say, I need to see Doctor. He say, "What happened? You have to go out today." Then, after, it was coming back good. But that's the time, 1984, we had the drought. It was so hot. We never had fan in the ward yet. Nothing. And then the people above us closed all their window, closed their door. And when the front door closed, no more air come through. So I was so desperate to keep cool, I went under the shower and stayed under the shower in the cold water. And some of the water came in my eye. Next day it got infected. The doctor told me he think I'm gonna lose my right eye. It was hurting me,. The pain was so excruciating. He send me to another doctor. He look at that, he said, "We have to remove that. Otherwise it's gonna hurt this left eye." So they took it out. Then when I came home, my husband set over there, we were having lunch. He look at me, he say, "Oh, my darling. Poor thing, my darling." Cause I never had eye. I should have gotten glass eye, and they could fix it a little better. After ten years I went back to try that. They said cannot. Too late. It's grown out of proportion already. That's why my eye stay like this. I get cataract on this left eye too. But they told me my eye wasn't strong enough to take the implant, so I couldn't have. I was just a loser. I can see only a little.

Why I wear hat, I wear hat to stop them from staring at me like a freak. [Because she has no eye on the right side, Cathrine wears a visor day and night so that people cannot see that it is missing.] And too, the glare of the sun hurts my eye. I tried to go to church without it, but someone stared at me. My husband told me to put it back on. Sometimes visitors at church try to get close to me and look under my visor. I can tell. I get angry when people stare at me. When I see disabled people, I avoid looking at them. I look away, because it's rude to stare. I wear the visor to protect myself from being stared at. I get one drawerful, it's just full of visors. You know, I was always lucky to get a perfect match with my clothes, to find something to match. Sometime people wonder why I wear hat at night. So I get the glitter ones. It kinda goes with your outfit, yeah?

Patients should be equal. But the patients look down on the next one if they're better looking, or whatever. Not enough we have that word leprosy on us, we have to be disfigured. That's why people scared of us. You see, one day I went with Katherine Costales. And Katherine is still clean. She never had it like us. And this lady came in our church hall, she told Katherine, "You are beautiful." And you know, that made me feel so bad that I didn't come up to Katherine, I didn't look like Katherine. It hurt me so bad I cried. I was angry. Because she looked good, they say, "You are beautiful." She had leprosy, but she was one of the lucky one that didn't get disfigured. That makes us very unhappy. People don't know how they can hurt us by distinguishing the pretty from the ugly. Yeah? It's not fair. I said, "Why should I suffer any more? How much more can we be punished? How much more can we be punished?

So I don't know, I feel like God left us to be something to show the people, that's what can happen to us. I just feel left behind, because I think he know who can handle it. It's sad you know. I wish I were beautiful, but I'm not. Sometimes I get so upset, why I have to be the one left behind, to show people what it is to be a leper. All the other guys, he took 'em home already, but he left us here to be witness. He let us be lepers. I think he thought maybe we could handle it. There's a lotta people killed themself, because they cannot handle. I will never kill myself.

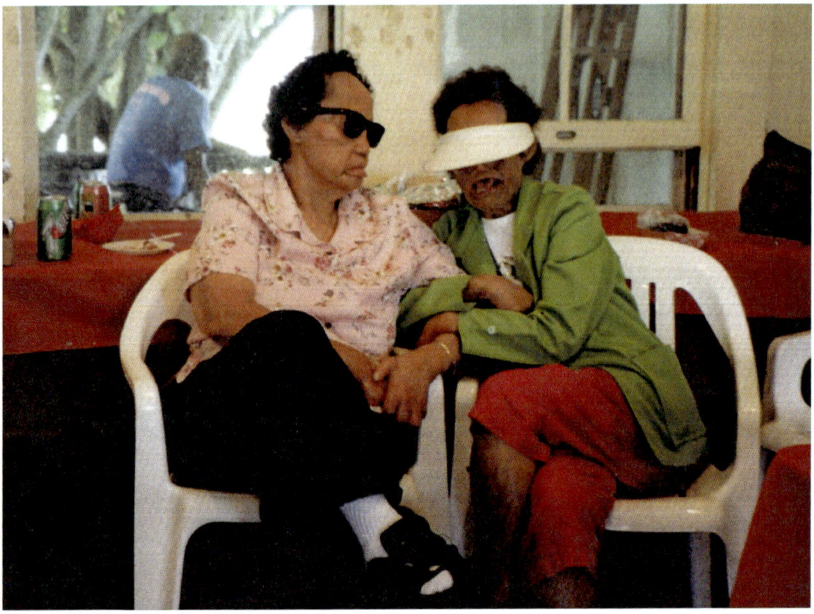
Cathrine and Lucy, c. 2006, "Still here."

And every time I tell Lucy—she and I the last girls from the Bishop Home bunch—"You and I are still here." And we hold each other's hand. I say, "We still here." All the girls that died, they looked good. They had beautiful noses, they had beautiful faces; but they all died. So I tell Lucy, "Look at us. We still here."

Hale Mohalu Struggle (1978-1983)

[In 1977, the State of Hawai'i decided to close the patient facility at Hale Mohalu in Pearl City. The patients objected and some of them refused to move out, even after water and electricity to the facility were turned off. Finally, the last patients were carried out by the police in 1983.]

It started 1979. Hale Mohalu was considered a home away from home. When we go back for the doctor's checkup, that is where we like to stay. Not to live, but we needed a second home where we can go there and just stay one week, two week and there's a place for us.

So, I think that's what made me think, if we lose that, where we going stay? And the rooms at Hale Mohalu are nice. Nothing fancy, but comfortable. And then we had the bathroom in between of another bedroom. And that we liked. We didn't like the commune kind. Yeah? We like privacy. So that's why we wanted to keep Hale Mohalu at Pearl City.

And we don't know it's gonna be [moved] up Leʻahi. They never talk about that place yet. We thought would be Waimanu Home or Kaneʻohe. And all this thing could have been avoided if the governor and the lieutenant governor had spoke to us about what's gonna happen. We would have never fight the issue. Never. They just told us to "Trust us." We cannot trust everybody, you know. And they keep telling us, "Trust us." What we thought, they was gonna make a second park. They had one further down, Pearl City Park. So we didn't wanta give this place up for another. After, way after everything happened, we found out that they was gonna get that place ready for low income housing, for sick people that they don't have a home and other handicapped people. If they had told us what they had planned to do, we would have never fought them. We'd have let go and come home. Because we think that is a good idea what they did. You know? Get somebody else living too and looking for a place to stay. But they didn't tell us. They think we don't have to know.

For the likes of me, I don't know how I got involved. It's the first time I ever did something like this. I never even thought I would be caught up in something like this. I just happened to be around some people when they were talking and that got me upset. So I kinda join in, and kind of talk with them, and go along with them, you know. And pretty soon I was deeply involved and I couldn't come back. I just felt that I have to keep on going. And they took away everything from us—the nurses, the food, the electricity, the water. Took everything away from us. But there were nice people that help us. We had a lotta supporters. And today they're still around, waiting for something else to happen, so they can support. You know, everybody has the right to think and do what they think is right. Even if you lose, at least you took a stab at it. You know? Just don't sit back and say, "Oh, they don't know what they doing." Get involved! Even if you lose, at least you stepped forward to help them.

Some patients supported us—they sent food. Some of them thought we were troublemakers; they didn't want any part of it. When we came back they said, "How come you folks wanted to make so much trouble with the government?"

Over there at Hale Mohalu we had Mary and Frank, they were husband and wife. And she happened to be a dialysis patient. But she came there, and she one of the diehard, you know. She say, "I'm gonna stay with you folks. I'm not leaving." And then her husband too, he help us a lot. And there were Bernice and Richard Pupule, they another diehards too. They supported everything that we did. And there was Suzuko and Sacadraca, husband and wife. She's Japanese and he was Filipino. But we all was going for the same cause. Then there was my husband. What we would do was, I come down two weeks. Then I go back Kalaupapa two weeks, my husband come down two weeks, then go back. See, we had to keep our yard down. The grass grow fast. So that's why my husband and I were going back and forth, to take care of our yard, our house, and we had animals. But we always went back to help out. And there was Winifred and Paul Harada, they were there too to support us in any way they could. And Boogie, he never go down with us, but he was always supporting us. He send us fish, you know, things like that.

And Bernard [Punikai'a] was our leader. He was so smart. He knew how to deal with those people. He knew how to talk. He knew a lotta well-known people, and got in touch with them for help. And they all came, supported us all the way. And our governor [Ariyoshi] never liked that. See, some was Republicans, some were Democrats, you know? Ariyoshi [Republican] didn't like what Abercrombie [Democrat] was doing. Abercrombie supported us. He carried signs, you know, that he made. He put the paper or cardboard on the floor.

They said go ahead, and start writing what you think is right. And you gonna carry this in front of the Washington Place, the capitol, where Ariyoshi was. So we all carrying signs on the sidewalk. Abercrombie find out Ariyoshi had his group out there too. Ariyoshi was running for office. We walk with our sign, and they walk. And then we just give them the eye. And they look at us, we try to go close to them, they giving us scared-eye look, you know. But we stayed there until sundown doing our part, carrying sign all day. And then we sit down in a group, somebody wen make lunch for us. And then the cars would pass by, our supporters, and they tooted the horn, you know? We had a lotta help from different people. And that was almost every other day we went to the capitol and do the same thing. To me was fun.

One time Ariyoshi came to Hale Mohalu. He had bodyguards with guns. The police thought we had guns. But we wasn't going to go that far. He came early, about 7:30, 8:00. It was Sunday. He wanted to catch us off-guard. So. And I hear people talking, I open my door, stick my head out. I close the door, I say, "Hey, honey, the governor coming." He said, "What? The governor?" And then I can see the gun sticking out, just like anybody jump for the governor, they shoot 'em. So, they went around and then they wanted to meet with all us. So we stood on the step, and they stood down, and the gun handle was still showing. Like anybody make a move, they was going shoot. He tell us go home. He came down to tell us go home Kalaupapa. We said, "No, we like live down here. We like keep this place for our second house, a place to stay."

And you know when we was down there at Hale Mohalu, we used to see these people sneaking around by the window. And then we went outside there, "What the hell you guys doin over here? Who are you?" And you know who they were? Channel 4, channel 2, channel 9. We said, "You folks like talk to us, come right in. Come right in and ask us all the question you like." And they came in. And they said they sorry, you know, because they thought us would chase him away. "Oh no, what you guys like ask? Just ask us, we tell you." So we tell 'em what we was fighting for.

And then, got hotter and hotter—by 1980. And that's when they used force on us. They cut the electric off, they cut the water off. And when they came to shut off the electricity? The guy was on the post, and Clarence [Naia, one of the patients], he say, "How come you like do like this to us? We no more light." He say, "If I don't do like this, they going kick me off my job." You know, they talk like that, eh? So we said, "God, now what we gotta do? Use flashlight?" They said, "You know, I sorry this happen, but that's my job. I gotta do what they tell me do." But our supporters brought us flashlight. Then we had so much supporters. So many of them gave up their time. After that they shut the water. Then Mayor Fasi went step in. Mayor Fasi brought us a big tank wagon water. When we like water, we go out fill up our bucket, put 'em in our room. You know, for take a shower or whatever. And then Ariyoshi and him got into a big fight. "Oh, he's looking for people vote for him, that's why he down there." No, I think Fasi really felt bad for us. Things were just going… cut off the light, cut off the water. And they cut off the food. We never had kaukau. But the supporters brought us food. They brought us kaukau every day. And they brought us blankets. And then on Saturdays, they got big shindig down there. All the supporters from all over come. Even my cousins, they come down. They tell me, "How? You like knock off anybody?" I say, "No, no, no, not that kind. We no like that kind. We like do it the nice way. You know? Just run 'em down. But we never like knock off anybody." "Oh, okay. You get anybody knock off, you call us up." "No, no, I no like go that far."

They carried Bernard and Clarence out. All the girls went home cause they were saying that they was going to send the bulldozer. They didn't want us around when that was gonna happen, when the building was gonna be crush. You know. That was Ariyoshi. He the one wen hit that place. Even the policemen, they carrying somebody out, and he saying, "Hey brah, you know I get Hawaiian, you get Hawaiian." "Yeah, but you know, that's where I get pay check." They was so scared. If they did not do what they supposed to do, they going fire them. You know? So they did what they were told to do.

And then they told us the sad news. Because they said that the bulldozer finally came out and they just rap the building. With toilet and basin inside, they just smash everything. They didn't wait to take out the basin, you know, the toilet. They just smash everything. I think that was an awful waste. They get plenty people that's so poor, they'd like to use that toilet.

They was wrong for not inviting us in on this plan that they had, to make it into a old folks home. I don't say Ariyoshi was all bad. He was a good governor. But he should have involved us, talked to us. We can listen. We are human beings. We have the right to know what's coming, what's gonna happen. Treat us as such. That's why I hate when doctors talk to the nurse about my condition. They don't think I'm smart enough to talk. I get upset. I just tell 'em, "Talk to me. I can answer you. I know what you talking about." They say, "Oh." You see, they don't trust us. That's because they think we don't know enough. I learned a lot in all the years in Kalihi. You learn to talk with people, and you learn to reason with people. You know? That's what you learn to do. Speak up. Don't sit down and say nothing. Later on you sorry.

Others at Kalaupapa, they just wanted to be quiet and let the bosses know that they were good patients, they're not troublemakers. But if you don't ask for things, you will not get anything. They think you satisfied with what you have. But there are other things that coming in, something new, you like to try that part of life. Some they never fight. All the rest of the patients get angry, because what they give us, she's gonna get too. She never helped fight, but she's gonna get it. We like everybody help out, speak up.

Work and Crafts

I was jack of all trades. I was a janitor, I was a dish washer, I worked in the dining room. And I cleaned yard. Oh, and orderly too—handling bed pans and all. Oh, I did lotta jobs, here and there. I worked for the blinds. They hard to work with, cause they can be very fussy, yeah? But I work there [at Bay View Home]. I work at the big dining room. And there were young guys up there, very cocky, you know. We had to take all that what they say.

And then I had to finish my work. So I work some down Hale Mohalu, and they added that on to what I had Kalaupapa, and I had my pension. 1972 I had my pension. And then Jubilee was pension 1973. They say you just gotta go on twenty years, you don't have to work for them any longer, and then we have pension. Now, if we had gone one more year, our pension would have jumped up. But I couldn't wait to get out of that job. I was tired of washing dishes. I was tired of mopping up. You know? I just needed to satisfy myself, get out of it, so we could sleep late. I didn't think about later on.

I used to sew a lot when I had good eyes. I never took lessons. It's almost still like my mother was with me. My mother did the sewing at home; I didn't. But I wanted to, so I sewed. I made muʻumuʻu's for myself, nice kine. Then I said, "Oh, I wanna go farther than that." I made a muʻumuʻu for my mother-in-law and a shirt for my father-in-law. And I never made shirts before. Things just like was coming to me for just a little while. So while I could do it, I used to sew up until 1:00 in the morning. I stop only to cook supper and then I go right back to my sewing. And then one day, it just left me. I just didn't wanna do it anymore. I cannot understand how I could do things before. I dunno how it came to me. Who was teaching me? I only can think, oh it could be my mother or my grandmother. My grandmother used to sew the hand kine, simple style. And I loved it and I made one exactly like how she made for me when I was six years old—same material. I bought the material, I cut the pattern the same, and I wore the dress and I felt like "Oh, I used to wear something like this before, when I was small." So it just took me back to the early years. You know? It was a simple pattern. Behind, it was just straight, down to my knees. And in front, it was straight to my waist. Then I add another piece of material with pleats only in the front. And I did it the same way my grandmother did. So I think that my mother and my grandmother—there was a force. The two of them gave me the power like, to sew. But almost like it was for a short time, you know? Grasp what you can right now cause you gonna lose it quick, yeah? That's what happened. When I put my sewing machine away, I never took it out again—'til today.

I love to cook. I LOVE to do crafts. I dunno why. It keeps me going. Crafts were just like part of my life. Before we had so much shells on the beach. And my girlfriend, she and I start picking up. We put in a box, load them up. There's nobody before us had anything like this in their mind, to do craft work. So it was left on the beach, tons and tons of shells. Nobody care. But when we had this craft, we went down the beach and pick them all up and we made things out of the shells and sold them and made some money. Good money. One year we made thousand dollars. And when they heard about what we was doing, they went down the beach with the kind—just like rake—to find all the shells. Today, there's hardly anything down there. Lucky if you can find one leho [cowry] shell.

Oh, we just had fun doing those things. The whole settlement was eying us up. And we sold lunch plates. The kokuas like that—with the baked beans with hot dog and buns, and one big piece chicken, and potato salad. They no go up the kitchen eat. They come down our place and ask 'How much your plate lunch?" "$4." "I like two." We made good money out of the lunch plates. The kitchen get stuck with their food. They come to us and they said, "No make kaukau – the kind 'ono kine [tasty kind]. Nobody come eat." I said, "Serve them supper." We let them go inside—you know, get soda and anything to bring them on. And then they go look and I say, "It opens 10:00." 10:00, the door fly open. Everybody inside they grabbing, and grabbing. They pay. That night when pau, we count and make about $400 - $500. Good. Then we make another one again – another $500.

Sarah always told us don't collect sticks and stones, because some stones are cursed. She always told us not to pick up sticks. Said the odd-looking sticks or odd-looking stones, don't bring it home. She said sometimes people worship them, and when they die it just get left like that. If you pick it up, it's going to follow you around. So we pick up shells, coral, you know, away from the bushes. And if we did pick up a stone from the bushes, we never tell Sarah. Because she going throw it away. But then we stay down Papaloa on the beach, get shells from the beach.

I had a lot of leho shells and most of the parts was broken off. It left only the lips, like. So one time I had twelve pictures on the wall--I wanted the frame. So what I did, I paint the picture all the same color—solid color. Then I put the leho lips—the small lehos—I made two eyes. Then the coral shell, it goes to a point, I made that as a nose. And the big lip I made—shape like a lip—I put it for the lip. Then I added seaweeds for the hair. And you know, I put it on my wall and my husband said, "Eh, where you got that from?" I said, "I made that." He said, "Eh, looks nice." So I had it on the wall in the hallway down by the door. I put it there purposely so when I get visitors, that's the first thing they going see. And I left the light on so they get better view.

Every time I get new ideas. Just like this last Christmas, we had a contest, I won first prize. So I tell my friend Jennifer, "I wanna do this one, the driftwood as a Christmas scene, a manger scene." She said, "Oh. You think you can get enough things for all that?" I said, "Yeah." So she said, "Okay." But before I did this, you know I was going to Las Vegas, so we stop at the shops for shells and they have all kinds of shells. And I got all the right shells for my three wisemen, my three kings, and for Joseph and Mary and I had a cute shell for baby Jesus. It was iridescent. And the shell that I used for his crib came from China. And I had other shells that I had before. Mary had a shell over her head like a halo and Joseph had one, too. They were stooping over the baby Jesus. It was beautiful. And I had two holes drilled. I had two red candles inside. I just threw little glue here and there and a little glitter and it turned out to be so beautiful.

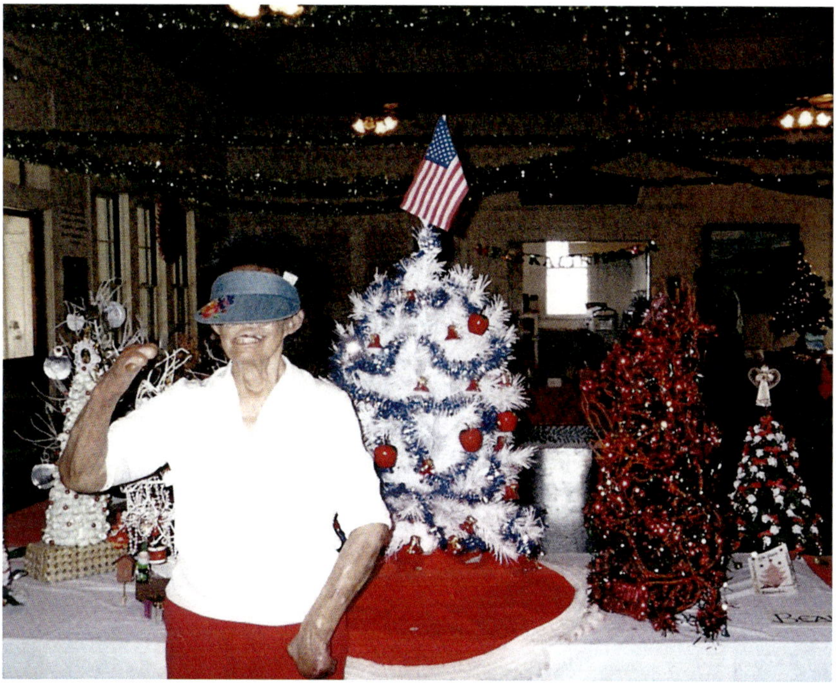

Cathrine with Trees Crafted for the Festival of Trees.
(photo by Ka‘ohulani McGuire)

I predicted my other one was gonna win, too. It was a dry Christmas tree frond and I wanted it to be natural, nothing with beads or sequin, just natural. So I had a hole drilled in one of the wood that I cut. I put this dry frond inside and then I cover it with Spanish moss—we call that hinahina. So I put it all up—it was high, but it didn't look right. So I grabbed the back of it, I snapped it. I bend it down little bit so the tree was short and look like the hinahina was overloading the tree and it naturally cracked and bend over because of the weight. When the judges came in, I was sitting there already. You know, away from the things. The judge came in, he was Japanese. Lucky thing was Japanese. Hawaiians wouldn't see anything—they just get the blinders on. The Japanese came inside. He said all he saw was that gray, and he said, "Oh my! Oh my!" He went right up to my tree and he told Ellen [the woman in charge of the contest], "This is very beautiful—so natural. First prize!" Oh, I was so happy. I had two first prize.

Work with IDEA (1997-2004)

[IDEA, International Organization for Integration, Dignity and Economic Advancement, was founded to work for the human rights of Hansen's Disease patients by Anwei Skinsnes Law, currently the international coordinator. Besides Cathrine, Kalaupapa patients Olivia Breitha and Bernard Punikaia were long involved in the work of IDEA.]

I got involved by accident. I was not in the group. I heard about it, but nobody asked me if I wanted to join. They was supposed to take Olivia to Spain. Olivia wasn't feeling good. She thought that it was too long—two weeks. So Anwei called my house. She told me, "Are you interested in takin a trip with the IDEA? I says, "Where?" She said, "To Spain." I said, "Oh, too far. I don't know." She said, "You talk it over with your husband." I went to talk with him and he said he don't wanta go. I said, "No, they askin me. But if you wanta go you can pay your own trip and go with us.." He didn't wanta go. So I went to Spain for two weeks. I saw a lotta things I would never see otherwise, before I go blind.

In Spain we went on this train. Go all over where you like go. And we went to have dinner at 10:00 at night. We got through eating at 2:00 in the morning all the time. And we sleep all through until twelve I think. The best hotel I like was Valencia. Beautiful hotel. After that, we went to the place we came for, Frontier. That's a leper colony. It was taken care by the Catholic priests and the nuns. By the time we went, there were just a handful of patients. And we went because they was tryin to close up all the leprosarium that they had. They said that the state would take care of the place if they allowed other chronic diseases in, like people with cancer, with tuberculosis, and AIDS. What we went to do was to talk to the patients, cause everybody's so confused. Until the people that live in there accepted the fact that there're gonna be other people put in with them so the state will take care of them. We went there to support them and that made it easier, they all just like agreed to it. They don't have to be sent out.

I'm glad I went. Because the patients on the other side didn't know about us. And we went up, and we stood on a stage, and we talked. We talk about our handicap, we talk about how we live here, and they all enjoyed listening to the ladies. You see they [IDEA] used to take only the men. The men hardly talk. So, Anwei told me, "Cathrine, talk to them about what you went through, and all that." And they all clap. And the ladies look at us, they feel happy that not only them are disfigured, get somebody else with the same problem. So we came friends. And then they hug us, and we hug them back.

Then I went to China two weeks. We stayed in Beijing for one week. We did everything in Beijing—Forbidden City, the five temples, and the Great Wall.

Anwei said the doctors are paid free trip to China, to go on this job to work with the people with Hansen's disease—to talk with them, and get to know them, and tell them about the new medicine and all that. And she said, "Let's go check them out, how they can get free money to go to do this job. Sometimes I feel they don't go to the meeting." Sure enough. We went to the meeting. Sometimes they have over fifteen doctors supposed to visit this meeting. Had only about three or four. The rest was on excursion.

When we went to see the people in the leprosarium in China. They were living at the end of the road. That's where you find all this kind hospitals, at the end of the road. I went in the front. They look at me, and they happy to see me. They know I get the sick. They see my hands and my face, and they happy that not only them have that problem, there's others too. So, they got friendly. They don't speak English; they talk in Chinese. We had a translator with us. Was a nice visit. They made lunch for us. Oh, man, we had a very good lunch. They cook vegetables. We had all kinda good food. We had nice time with them. Then it was time for us to say goodbye. They all come to us. Hug us. And the word they give us, "Sheh-sheh." Thank you.

Chapter 5. Getting Old

Death of Jubilee (1997)

I went to Spain—that's when my husband died. I came home, I was at Hale Mohalu, when I heard them whisper. I heard the nurse say, "Oh, he's gone already." But I never pay attention. I was too tired. It was a long trip, you know.

But before I went, we had a checkup—thorough checkup, blood, everything. Doctor said me and Jubilee are good, no problem. Within two weeks he died. I was angry with Doctor. I said, "Doctor, you checked everything, our tests. You say we are good. How come he's dead?" Doctor couldn't answer me. But something was wrong with him. They say that my husband died from a stroke. So, they left it at that. He's dead already. I couldn't do anything about it, but I blame myself for leaving him. You see, my husband, sometime when he sleep he don't breathe. And, you know, if I don't hear him breathe, I go in his room, I bang the bed, and he start up. I gotta hide quick because he going get mad with me. But I do that because I don't hear him breathing. So I think that's how he died. I wasn't there to help him. I wasn't home the last two weeks for him to complain to me, and tell me, "You know, honey, there's something wrong with me." I was away, so he had nobody to talk to. And he will never go to nobody to tell them something's wrong with him. So he stayed like that. And just, one night, when he fell asleep, then it start happening, that his brain never tell him to breathe, and he died in that way. But he knew I was coming home. Like he wanted to stay alive to see me again.

So, I don't know. They were omens that I had in Spain. Valerie and I were standing under the tree. This big falcon dropped. I say, "What was that?" She say, "Oh, it's just an old dead bird." I say, "Oh no. That's a bad omen for me." It was right in front of me, a dead bird.

I say, "Oh no, something is wrong. Every time a dead bird show up, something is wrong."

So when we got back to America, I feel that's the time my husband died. 2:00 in the morning [in Hawai'i]. Doctor told me, "What makes you feel like he died 2:00?" I say, "Well, in New York, I was sleeping. When I got up I had a bad dream. I dreamt about my uncle who died long time ago. And Jubilee was his favorite." And I told them that he must have heard somebody say Jubilee was coming, you know, to go up there? And he was looking around, I guess, if he heard right. And I look at him and I say, "Uncle, what happened? What's the matter?" Didn't know what the answer, because I just see him in my dream. I got scared, you know, I got up and I stayed up. I didn't want to go back sleep. And the others say, "What's wrong?" I say, "I had a bad dream. Something is wrong. I don't know what, but something is wrong."

So we went down the airport, and then caught the plane, we came home. And I had to stay at Hale Mohalu, because we got in late. And the plane [for Kalaupapa] is not until next day. And my husband died 2:00 Sunday morning. Nobody knew about it until 5:00 in the afternoon. My husband was still soft yet when I came home, his hands was flexible. He's supposed to be hard already. That never set in yet. I said, gee, maybe if somebody gave him artificial respiration, maybe this wouldn't have happened. Cause when they brought his breakfast, he didn't get it. It was [still] in the box.[25] They brought lunch, he didn't get it, cause he's still in bed. When the boy brought supper, that's when he said, "Gee. How come this guy no eat all day?" It was Earl, so he said he go look if the car stay. The car still in the garage. And he go get the nurse, go up the house. They break in. He was dead on the bed. 2:00 that morning. They never find him till 5:00. He was dead fifteen hours.

They kept him all night at the meat house. Without telling me.

---

[25] Meals are delivered to a box that can be opened from outside the patient's house.

You know, it's no good you leave a body unattended. Hawaiians don't believe in that. All kind evil spirits going around, they all like go in the body, you know? I was kinda upset. I call the night nurse, I said, "Where is my husband?" You know what they told me? "I don't know where." I say, "How come you don't know where? You the night nurse. You supposed to know where everybody is." Then I put two and two together, I figure they get him down the ice house. I know. And that's what they did. They covered him up, all with the sheet. And they put him on the table. By himself. Before, we used to put in our church hall, and we have members of the church sit with them until next day. We never leave a body unattended. The members are down there all night. I was pretty upset.

They took him there the night before, and then the next day they put clothes on him and they put him in the church. But see, Kahu [the minister] don't know what we used to do before. He's a different age from us. I was surprised he wasn't the one that held my husband's body back. He was gonna let them bury my husband, without me seeing him. Albert Pu was the one. Albert said, "No way you guys gonna put him down. His wife is in Honolulu. You folks hold him till she come home." That's how they kept him. I thanked him. At least I got to kiss him goodbye. Oh, would be awful if I didn't see him, to say goodbye. He was just like sleeping. But I went by him, say "Honey." Just hoping he would say, "What?" But he was sleeping, he was gone. I just wanted to hug him and hold him.

The hospital, the nurses clean him up, and put clothes on him. They took him down to the church. I told 'em he didn't wanta be buried in the good clothes, he like jeans and t-shirt. "Oh yeah? he's lotta nice shirt." I say, "I'm doing what he wants. We talked about death." So some people no understand, just like I wanted him to go like that. That was his last request. Jubilee say, "I like one jeans and old t-shirt. I don't like nice shirt, nothing. Just bury me like that." Then I showed him the clothes I wanted to be buried in. I say, "This one." He said okay. Not knowing that death was right around the corner.

And I told him, "I don't think I'll ever want to get married." You know, we was talking about all this kind stuff. He tell me, "Why?" I said, "Because I love you so much, I cannot get married to anybody else." He say, "Well, you do what you want." We talk about that about three weeks before it happened. Maybe sometime it's good to talk about death, but sometime, you gotta be careful what you ask for. You know? there's somebody listening. You gotta be careful what you ask for, because you might get it. So I say, "Maybe it was wrong for us to talk about death. Don't talk about death in your house. Just talk about life."

Then at the church I was sitting down, then I saw the coffin cover move. So I said, I better go up and kiss my husband for the last time. I got up, I walked to the coffin. I bent over, I kissed my husband. Somebody came get me, take me back to the chair. I got so mad. They treated me like a child, like I couldn't think for myself. I thought they was gonna cover him up, I gotta give him the last kiss. You know? But no, they just took the cover away, and then we went on with the service. And then, after that, they said that if anybody want to view the body, to go up now. So, they had a lotta people go up. I didn't go up again. It'd be hard for me. I wouldn't wanta let go.

And you know when they cover the coffin, they took him out, and they put me and my family in the car, went down the graveyard. And I always feature before, if my husband was down in the coffin, I gonna scream my head off and yell. But that day I kept to myself. I didn't wanta do what other women did—scream for their husband. Three months after that they get married again. I didn't wanta do that. I just wanted to say goodbye to my husband, and remember all of the good times we had. Good fun times—what we did, where we went. And I loved every minute of it. I just was so sad it had to happen that way.

I don't know, I just think it was the hand of God. Because if I was home, then would get hard time take me away from my husband. I would hang on him. They would have to pry me loose. I don't think God will like me to do that. So I think he took Jubilee the way he did.

He knew how much I love my husband. I love him very much. And He made it a little easy for me. That's what I think.

I think death was around the corner for my husband. When I told the doctor that he died, he just look at me, like he had a hunch that my husband will die anytime now. Jubilee was acting strange toward that time. But I didn't get the message. I should have caught on what was happening. When I sang the songs that he brought to Kalaupapa, and he looked at me, I said, "Remember this song?" He said, "No." I said, "How can you forget? You brought it to Kalaupapa." I sang another one, I said, "Do you remember this one?" It seems like he lost track, like things was changing for him already. He kinda forget all those things.

My granddaughter was here a couple a weeks after Jubilee died, and she heard him walking in the living room. (She was in the front bedroom and I was in the back.) She said, "Who's that?" I said, "It's just your grandfather." He came back because he left something undone. He wanted to take care of me. Now I'm sorry I didn't go say something to him. I wanted to tell him, if I did anything wrong to forgive me. Because I wasn't here when he died. They [the spirits of the dead] cannot talk to us, because they've seen things that we not supposed to know about. But they can hear what we say.

Like Puna, [a woman whose husband had just died], every chance she gets she go down the grave, clean the grave, and she sit and talk story with him. We all do that. I go down the grave too. I talk to my husband. And I don't care if they leave me alone, because that's all I have. When I pau talk story I come home. After a while I let go. I didn't do it too long, cause people talked to me. They said, "You have to let him go. Because he's no longer with us, only his spirit, but he needs to go. Let him go." Now I just go down, say, "Hello honey, how you?" And I say, "I'm fine. Don't worry about me. I'm okay. And I still love you. So, I gotta go now. Rest in peace." Then I go.

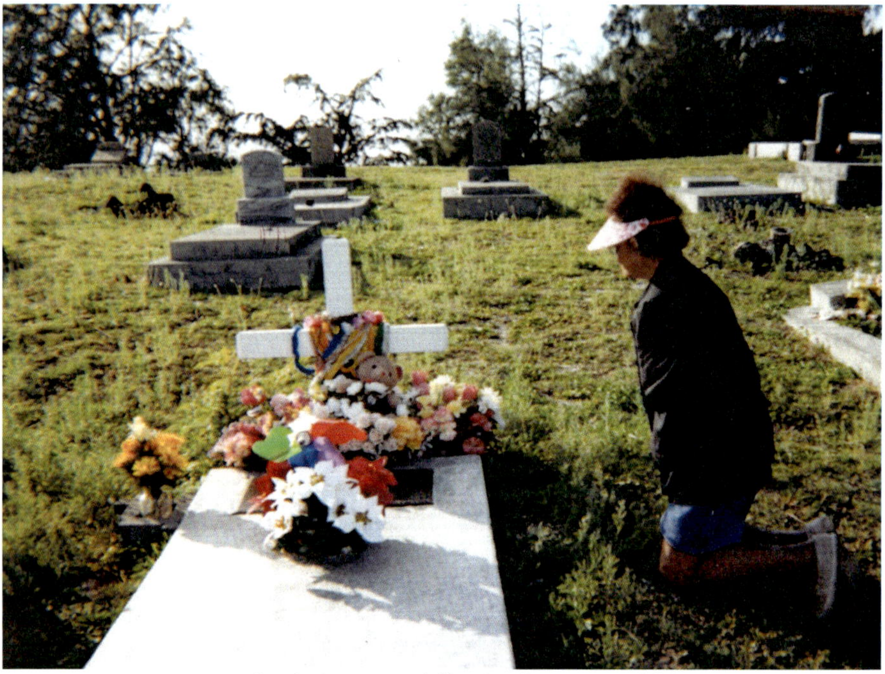

Cathrine at Jubilee's Grave, c. 2005.
(photo by Ka'ohulani McGuire)

You know it's seven years [in 2004]. Oh, I gotta go put flowers on my husband's grave. I don't wanta forget that I have a loved one there. I put flowers. I remember him every Christmas, cause before, every time I decorate the Christmas tree, he go down the bar, have three beers. When he come home, oh, he's so happy, tell me, "Oh honey, that looks nice." You know, the tree all decorated. And I get gifts under the tree. And I always feel, even he died, I put flowers on his grave. So I put poinsettias, a Christmas wreath, and I always feel like he's looking at me, and says, "Oh, I'm so glad you never forget me." I think about things like that, because it makes me happy, even though he's seven years dead. This April makes seven years. April 20.

Old Age

(2002)

I dreamt of Alice [a patient who has passed on] last night. I don't know how come. I was going up Bishop Home for something. And then I was coming down the road where my car was park on the left side, and Alice pass me. She didn't look at me but she was looking at the cat that was in my car. And she was making motion like, to the cat. Mew, Mew. And Alice was look young yet, you know? Not sickly, she look good. But she didn't say anything to me. Sometime it's good. You know, if she said something to me and I answered, I may have an early death. You know, just like I responding to her call, yeah? Cause many times [in dreams] I see the people that pass away and they say, "You wanna come?" Like they telling if I like go swimming and I dunno, sometime in me, I just hold back, I say, "No." And then they disappear. So always I fear if I going say, "Yeah." Just like I wanna join them. I don't wanna join them yet, I'm not ready. I'm not through with my work yet on earth. The only way I go is, God take me, I gotta go. But if I can help it, I want Him to know that I'm not ready yet. I want Him to know that I love life and I want to be here yet. I know if I go, I going be with my husband. You know? But if I not dead, I don't wanna think about that.

(2005)

See us, we don't know when the Lord going take us. Yeah? We don't know when. You just gotta be ready. Everybody say, "Lord, I'm not ready. I don't wanta go yet. Cause I almost died one evening about three years ago. My heart, I had too much fluid in my lungs. I could barely walk. So I just reach the porch, I open the door, I had to sit on the floor. Cause I was too knock out. I sat on the floor and I say, "Oh Lord, not yet. I not ready. I don't wanta go yet." I thought I was going. I tell Dr. Jones that, Doctor look at me, he said, "Well, you had water in your lungs. That's why you got tired." And he said, "You have to watch your water intake." Then he said, "How much beer do you drink? Do you drink beer?" I tell, "I love to drink." And he said, "Two bottle. Only two bottle." I said, "Beer?" He said, "Yes. What else do you drink?" I say, "I love wine." "Oh, one glass." He don't know I clean the whole bottle up. We come up the hall [for a party] and I drank 'em all. See, Doctor tell us things like that so we don't get carried away. But he forget, sometimes we go on our own. We no listen, eh? I say, Oh, Doctor lying to me. I think I can drink more than that. I gotta watch myself. I don't drink every time. I drink once in a while, but not every night. Sometime I don't go down the bar three, four months.

(2006)

Ghost town, that's what this place feels like. That should be the name of the book. Lot of people died. We feel the loneliness now, feel the emptiness.

You know, a lotta people think that getting old is beautiful. It's not beautiful. I have arthritis, I have eye trouble, I can't do what want to do. I say it's not beautiful, it's very lonesome. You don't have friends; you be a lonely, lonely person. But I have two friends that always come to look for me and take me to the bar, or we meet some place else—Gertrude and Elizabeth. I'm just a little older than them, but we like to do the same things. We know each other, how we feel. It is a very lonely thing to be by yourself. But if you learn to do things—like, I love crafting, and if I had my two eyes, it wouldn't be so bad. But because I'm losing my sight, just like, there's nothing left for me. What's the use of staying here? I might as well join my husband. Just being blind, you have to depend on people—to help you get your meals, help you clean your house. And then sometime they do a little more than that, they keep you company. And you know they are tired, they wanta go home. Some of them are really nice about that. I don't know. I'm seventy-nine, and sometime you feel like this could all be over, if you let it happen. Sometime you think about that. But I always tell God, "I'm not ready."

I always wanted to go to Japan. So Anwei [Coordinator of IDEA] came, and she saw me, and she say, "We're thinking about going to Japan [in Spring 2007]. Would you like to go?" I said, "Would I like to go? Yes." I always heard so much about Japan. I want to see where and how the patients live. I always think they live around a spacious area, where they can make their own garden, and have water running, and gold fish. The Japanese love to do things like that. And I like to see weeping willow trees hanging over. And I like to see the bridges that go up like that [arched], you know? I like to walk on those. And then I like to meet all the patient, the young people, the old people. What I would do is, I would go [demonstrates bowing]. To show some respect, yeah? I like to do things like that.

Afterword

The summer of 2007 was Cathrine's eightieth birthday and she had a party for the whole of Kalaupapa Settlement for her birthday. She loved it: "I'm so lucky. I had so much help making my party. They all offered, because they knew I cannot do nothing."

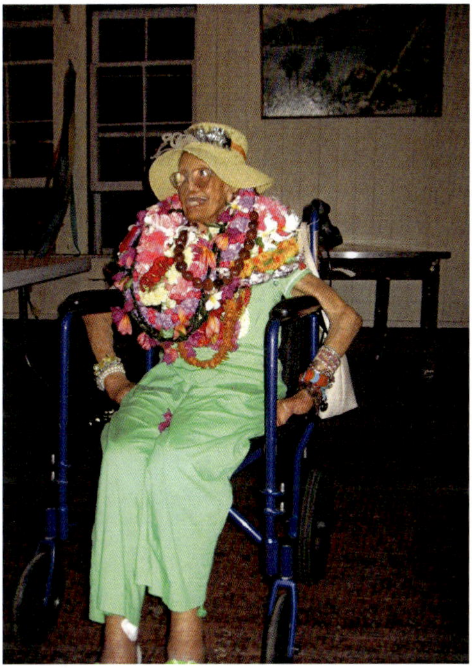

Cathrine on Her 80th Birthday
(photo by C. Langlas)

Many people had brought flower lei for her. And she loved her lei:

"I was ecstatic. I never had lei like that before. I never expected that. The nurses told me to take the lei off, because it's too hot and the smell is too strong, but I said no. They don't know I'm a Polynesian! I can take the heat and the flower smell. I know I'll never have lei like that again. I would stay like that, even if I'm hot."

Cathrine passed away in July 2008, just after her birthday in June. She had a premonition that death was near. When I called her in May to say that I was going to Europe on vacation and that I wouldn't come to Kalaupapa to see her until August, she told me that she might not live that long. I should have listened to her.

Appendix. Background on Kalaupapa

Kalaupapa Settlement Over Time

Kalaupapa Peninsula on the Island of Moloka'i was chosen for a Hansen's disease settlement by the Hawaiian Kingdom in 1865 because of its isolation. The only access to Kalaupapa by land was a steep trail down the cliff face (pali) from "Topside" Moloka'i to the south of the peninsula. The isolation of Kalaupapa made it seem like a prison in the early days. Under the Territory of Hawai'i, the Board of Health continued to run Kalaupapa Settlement as a place of confinement for patients with Hansen's disease. Today, those with Hansen's disease are no longer confined and Kalaupapa Settlement is run by the state for those who were formerly confined there who want to remain at Kalaupapa. There is an airfield and daily flights come in from Honolulu and from Topside Moloka'i. Kalaupapa is no longer difficult of access physically, but the State Department of Health (DOH) which runs Kalaupapa Settlement today still limits visitation by outsiders. Both the patients and the DOH workers describe Kalaupapa today as a refuge from the outside world. It is a place without hustle and bustle, without traffic noise, without violent crime. For the patients it is also a refuge in the sense that they don't need to worry about being stared at, if they have been physically altered by the disease. Nor do they need to fear being stigmatized and rejected when outsiders learn that they come from Kalaupapa.

When patients were brought to Kalaupapa in the 1940s their feelings were very different. Often they were brought against their will, having been torn away from their families. When they arrived they were confronted with patients in an advanced stage of Hansen's disease, and they saw in them their fate—alteration of the face, loss of fingers and toes, blindness, and in a few years death. Kalaupapa then was a prison to which they were consigned by the government of Hawai'i, to prevent their disease from spreading to others. The patients' sense of Kalaupapa has been transformed today, partly because they no longer are forced to remain at Kalaupapa, partly because they came to dread the outside world. The state's isolation policy was ended as a result of the introduction of antibiotic drugs which put the disease into remission. The first sulfone antibiotics were introduced in 1946, when the use of the drugs was still experimental, the dosage uncertain. It took about ten years for most patients before they were pronounced "inactive" (as determined by testing of body tissue for the bacteria) and were placed on "temporary release." Those on temporary release could leave Kalaupapa and get a job outside. In 1969, the state officially ended its program of forced segregation for those with Hansen's disease. Some of the Kalaupapa patients left after they were released, but many chose to stay. Those patients who moved out sometimes had a difficult time adjusting to the complications of life outside.

Prior to 1946, the Kalaupapa Settlement was in constant flux. Many patients died after they had been at Kalaupapa a few years. They were replaced by new patients from outsid. (Normally they spent a few years first at Kalihi Hospital on O'ahu, and were transferred to Kalaupapa when they disease became worse.) After 1949, the Board of Health set a policy that no new patients would be sent to Kalaupapa except at their request. After that patients would normally be treated at Hale Mohalu, a facility set up in Pearl City, O'ahu to replace Kalihi Hospital that was closed at that time. Up to 1969, a small number of patients at Hale Mohalu were allowed to transfer to Kalaupapa on request, but the number of new arrivals was small. After 1969, no new patients were admitted. The population of patients has gradually dwindled since 1969 as the patients get older and die.

In the 1940s when Cathrine came to Kalaupapa, most of the patients lived in one of four group homes built in the Settlement—Bay View Home, Bishop Home, Baldwin Home, and McVeigh Home.

Each of the homes had one or more dormitory buildings, a kitchen and a communal dining room. McVeigh Home also had a cluster of cottages for married patients. Bay View Home had a large proportion of blind or disabled men. Bishop Home was run by nuns of the St. Francis order. It was built to house blind and disabled women, but by the 1940s it housed more girls than older women. Baldwin Home was run by lay brothers of the Sacred Heart order and was established as a home for boys. (The original Baldwin Home was established at Kalawao and a new Baldwin Home was built at Kalaupapa when Kalawao was abandoned.) In addition, many married couples lived in houses outside the group homes. Each group home was a little community to itself, with its own dining regime and social life. The homes had their own baseball and volleyball teams that played other teams. As the number of patients dwindled, a larger proportion lived in individual houses and few were left in the group homes. By the late 1960s, the group home dining rooms were closed and many of the living rooms were given to kokuas to live in.

As the patients have aged they have become less able to take care of the work of the settlement and the proportion of non-patient workers in the community has increased. In the early 1960s most of the work of the settlement was being done by patients and they far outnumbered the non-patients who worked for the DOH. By 2002, the patients were outnumbered by non-patient workers. Only a few patients still work full-time today. The work of the Settlement itself is largely done now by DOH workers. In 1980, Kalaupapa Peninsula was made part of Kalaupapa National Historical Park, and there is now a sizable staff of federal workers at Kalaupapa as well.

Kalaupapa as a Place

Kalaupapa National Historical Park includes Kalaupapa Peninsula, together with the adjoining Waihänau, Wai‘ale‘ia and Waikolu Valleys. (See the map on the next page.) On the leeward (eastern) side of the peninsula is Kalaupapa Settlement proper, containing the residences of Kalaupapa patients and workers and the buildings occupied by the State Department of Health and the National Park Service. The leeward side of the peninsula has a sand beach, shallow water offshore and a broad reef. North of the settlement proper on the leeward side, is a large graveyard makai (seaward) of the road to the airport, in the area known as Papaloa. The graveyard is still in use for the burial of patients. Further north is a group of beach houses built and owned by patients and often used by them to house their visitors. The paved road ends at the airport, although there is a track that leads further, all the way around the peninsula. From the airport on east around the windward side of the peninsula there is no reef; the water at the shore is deeper and rougher. On the east side of the airport is the old lighthouse and the beach area called Hoʻolehua. At Hoʻolehua beach there are many saltwater ponds where salt is harvested in the summertime. The remainder of the windward coast of the peninsula is traveled mainly by fishermen and by visitors to Kalaupapa who are being shown "around the island" by their hosts.

A second road leads inland from Kalaupapa Settlement proper and east to Kalawao and Judd Park on the eastern side of the peninsula. Kalawao is the location of the old nineteenth century settlement for Hansen's disease patients. The patients were moved from Kalawao to the east side of the peninsula early in the twentieth century. Judd Park has a small pavilion used for picnics and a beautiful view of two small offshore islands. On the southwest side of the peninsula, where it tapers off, there is a long black sand beach. The beach is traversed by the trail used by Kalaupapa workers and tourists to travel up and down the pali.

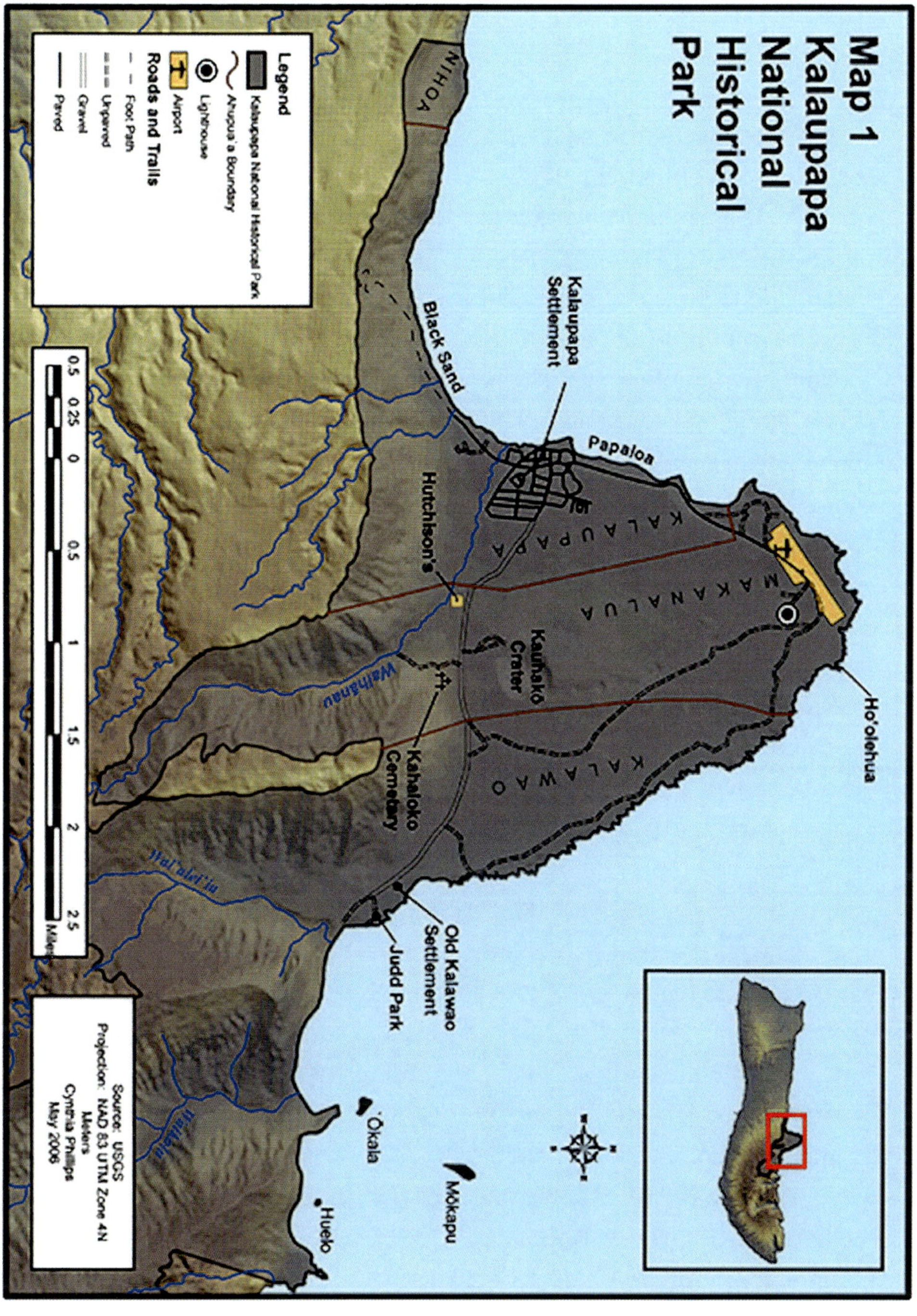
Map 1
Kalaupapa
National
Historical
Park
Legend
Kalaupapa National Historical Park
Ahupua'a Boundary
Lighthouse
Airport
Roads and Trails
Foot Path
Unpaved
Gravel
Paved
NIHOA
Black Sand
Kalaupapa Settlement
Papaloa
KALAUPAPA
Hutchison's
MAKANALUA
Kauhakō Crater
Ho'olehua
KALAWAO
Kahaloko Cemetary
Waihānau
Old Kalawao Settlement
Judd Park
Wai'ale'ia
'Ōkala
Mōkapu
Huelo
0.5 0.25 0 0.5 1 1.5 2 2.5
Miles
Source: USGS
Projection: NAD 83 UTM Zone 4N
Meters
Cynthia Phillips
May 2006

Patients and Kokuas

The most basic division at Kalaupapa is between patient and non-patient. Non-patients fall into two main categories, workers and visitors. At Kalaupapa, workers are commonly called "kokuas," both DOH workers and national park workers. The patients were brought to Kalaupapa to be isolated because they had Hansen's disease, and they have the right to reside at Kalaupapa as long as Kalaupapa Settlement is maintained by the state. The workers can only stay at Kalaupapa as long as they have a job with the State or the Park Service. Visitors are allowed to come in only for a limited time as guests of patients or workers, or as tourists who come for the day on the tour.

The term "kokua" derives from the past. Originally kokua was used for an individual without Hansen's disease who voluntarily accompanied a family member sent to Kalaupapa as a patient in order to help the patient. That was allowed during the nineteenth century and the early part of the twentieth century. The term comes from the Hawaiian word kōkua meaning "to help", or "helper." So, it originally meant one who came to help out of aloha, not as a paid worker. After a certain point, the Territory no longer allowed family members to come as kokuas. The term got extended to the Catholic nuns and lay brothers who cared for patients at Kalaupapa and to the state workers who were paid to care for patients. When the national park was established, the patients called the park workers kokuas as well, even though for the most part they do not directly care for the patients. Thus "kokua" has a sort of double meaning at Kalaupapa. It means "non-patient worker," but to local people who know the Hawaiian meaning it can also mean "someone who serves the patients."

Both patients and kokuas were part of the community during the period we stayed at Kalaupapa (2001-2008); and they all went to community parties. However, that was not the case in the past. In the days before segregation ended, there were many rules that limited contact between patients and kokuas, the most basic being that kokuas could not enter the house yard of a patient except as part of their work. The legacy of that separation remains today. Kokuas seldom visit patients at home today. Many patients are used to their privacy at home and many workers are unsure they would be welcome there.

Made in United States
North Haven, CT
05 November 2026

21766156R60073